Public Health in History

KU-624-436

WITHDRAWN

LIVERPOOL JMU LIBRARY

3 1111 01431 0294

Understanding Public Health

Series editors: Ros Plowman and Nicki Thorogood, London School of Hygiene & Tropical Medicine (previously edited by Nick Black and Rosalind Raine)

Throughout the world, there is growing recognition of the importance of public health to sustainable, safe and healthy societies. The achievements of public health in nineteenth-century Europe were for much of the twentieth century overshadowed by advances in personal care, in particular in hospital care. Now, with the dawning of a new century, there is increasing understanding of the inevitable limits of individual health care and of the need to complement such services with effective public health strategies. Major improvements in people's health will come from controlling communicable diseases, eradicating environmental hazards, improving people's diets, and enhancing the availability and quality of effective health care. To achieve this, every country needs a cadre of knowledgeable public health practitioners with social, political and organizational skills to lead and bring about changes at international, national and local levels.

This is one of a series of books that provides a foundation for those wishing to join in and contribute to the twenty-first-century regeneration of public health, helping to put the concerns and perspectives of public health at the heart of policy-making and service provision. While each book stands alone, together they provide a comprehensive account of the three main aims of public health: protecting the public from environmental hazards, improving the health of the public and ensuring high quality health services are available to all. Some of the books focus on methods, others on key topics. The books have been written by staff at the London School of Hygiene & Tropical Medicine with considerable experience of teaching public health to students from low-, middle- and high-income countries. Much of the material has been developed and tested with postgraduate students both in face-to-face teaching and through distance learning.

The books are designed for self-directed learning. Each chapter has explicit learning objectives, key terms are highlighted and the text contains many activities to enable the reader to test their own understanding of the ideas and material covered. Written in a clear and accessible style, the series will be essential reading for students taking postgraduate courses in public health and will also be of interest to public health practitioners and policy-makers.

Titles in the series

Forthcoming titles:

Public Health in History

Virginia Berridge, Martin Gorsky
and Alex Mold

 Open University Press

Open University Press
McGraw-Hill Education
McGraw-Hill House
Shoppenhangers Road
Maidenhead
Berkshire
England
SL6 2QL

email: enquiries@openup.co.uk
world wide web: www.openup.co.uk

and Two Penn Plaza, New York, NY 10121-2289, USA

First published 2011

Copyright © London School of Hygiene & Tropical Medicine 2011

All rights reserved. Except for the quotation of short passages for the purpose of criticism and review, no part of this publication may be reproduced, stored in a retrieval system, or transmitted, in any form or by any means, electronic, mechanical, photocopying, recording or otherwise, without the prior written permission of the publisher or a licence from the Copyright Licensing Agency Limited. Details of such licences (for reprographic reproduction) may be obtained from the Copyright Licensing Agency Ltd of Saffron House, 6–10 Kirby Street, London EC1N 8TS.

A catalogue record of this book is available from the British Library

ISBN-13: 978-0-33-524264-1 (pb)
ISBN-10: 0-33-524264-2 (pb)
eISBN: 978-0-33-524266-5

Library of Congress Cataloging-in-Publication Data
CIP data applied for

Typeset by RefineCatch Limited, Bungay, Suffolk
Printed in the UK by Bell & Bain Ltd, Glasgow

Fictitious names of companies, products, people, characters and/or data that may be used herein (in case studies or in examples) are not intended to represent any real individual, company, product or event.

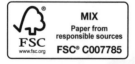

The *McGraw·Hill* Companies

Contents

List of figures

List of tables

Disclaimer

Every effort has been made to obtain permission from copyright holders to reproduce material in this book and acknowledge these sources correctly. Any omissions brought to our attention will be remedied in future editions.

Overview of the book

Introduction

In recent years, there has been much discussion about the role public health can play in improving health outcomes for populations. Much of this discussion takes place in the absence of a full understanding of the factors that led to the issues that now need to be addressed. The drivers of change and the impact of different motivating forces are overlooked. Sometimes the past is called upon to invoke a heroic public health figure, or to concentrate on a particular period, such as the mid-nineteenth century when sanitation was a major concern. Our purpose here is to show that the history of public health can provide a wider perspective on current policies and events. This wider history is beginning to be taught in schools of medicine and of public health. By making it available in this format, we hope to reach out to a broader audience and to those with little or no formal background in history.

This book provides an introduction to the history of public health in Europe, North America and the 'global South'. By the 'global South' we mean countries previously termed 'developing countries' and, prior to that, 'the colonies'. In several chapters readers will find that our discussion of public health in the West concentrates particularly on Britain. Britain has been chosen not only because many important developments in public health took place there, but also because it offers the opportunity to study specific issues in detail within one national context. By relating changes in public health in Britain to developments elsewhere in the world, we aim to explore how ideas, approaches and methods within public health differed from place to place and over time. Our time frame is primarily the nineteenth and twentieth centuries, the period when the precursors of modern public health systems and responses came into play.

Why study health history?

If you look at a television news programme, read a daily paper, or a news application, coverage of health issues is prominent: the consumption of alcohol or tobacco and their impact on health; sexual health or the spread of HIV/AIDS; and changes to the organization and funding of health services are among the news stories you might come across. Few days go by without health coverage.

This book integrates history into that relentless onslaught of health information and the concern about health statistics or health policy. We provide context for the here and now, and analysis of change over time. We examine the factors involved in making change happen, the alternative models, the roles of individuals, of social movements and of scientific theories in the process.

We often take the present for granted and assume that things have always been more or less as they are now. Looking at the past can make the present seem problematic and strange. Studying the past reveals that societies, policies and responses are not static and that things do change, and unveils some of the debates and alternative options available to people in the field at the time. There is a tendency, as we discuss in Chapter 1, to assume that human affairs have gone through stages of almost inevitable progress up to the present and to look at the past with a superior eye. Certainly many health indicators suggest that standards have improved for much of the world's population, but how that change has been achieved, and how and why particular issues have come on and off agendas, is worthy of study.

In this book, we examine the practical uses of history, something considered in detail in the final chapter of the book as well as in each topic chapter. But please bear in mind that all health issues and responses have their history, which may well have current significance both nationally and internationally. Take, for example, the controversial 'McKeown thesis', which argued that improvement in nutritional status due to rising living standards was the principal driver of improvements in population health in the modern era. This was used in global South countries in recent times to justify market-based policies for health. History was transferred into the present in a way that historians since then have disputed, something we discuss in Chapter 13. The study of history is not just about the establishment of past events, historical 'facts', it is a matter of interpretation and debate: we believe that the study of history, and an understanding of the debates and interpretations of the past, will help you if you wish to influence or work within public health in the present. Evidence is crucial to understanding health issues – and history is central to the discipline of history.

Structure of the book

In this book, 'public health' covers not just conventional historical meanings of the term, such as the nineteenth-century advances in water and sanitation or the early twentieth-century enthusiasm for health education and education for mothers. It also addresses health systems and service development, the rise of health professions and the role of gender in health and medicine. We also focus on a number of case studies – particular diseases or sets of activities (e.g. drug use) that have come to be seen within a public health framework in recent times.

The book begins with an introduction to the nature of history, to different schools of thought, and to sources and methods for its study. Overall, we see public health as an arena that has been subject to change; change both in the way in which it is defined and the activities that it is seen to cover. These changes define the framing of our book. In the nineteenth century, public health was a matter of the environment, of water and sanitation. In the latter years of the century, the advent and acceptance of germ theory brought a different form of public health, focused more on the role of the individual and on cleansing the individual environment. Further stages followed in the twentieth century – a public health focus on education and, after the Second World War, the rise of various forms of 'new public health', encompassing social medicine and leading to health promotion and primary health care. This framework shapes the core of the book, which is divided into three sections: the first deals with the nineteenth century; the second contains case studies that span the nineteenth and twentieth centuries; and the third concentrates on the twentieth century.

In Chapter 2, we begin our analysis of nineteenth-century public health, and examine the context for the emergence of public health as a movement and a concern in this period. Chapter 3 analyses the rationale for a response we now all take for granted – the role of the state. Why did states start to take public health regulation on board as part of their remit during these years? In Chapter 4, we look at the role of health professionals, and at the gendered division of health care labour, which has also affected the public health profession. In Chapter 5, we turn away from Britain and from Europe to examine the parallel rise of tropical medicine in the nineteenth century and its place within the expansion of Empire in the first decades of the twentieth century.

We then move on to examine a series of case studies that explore the development of particular public health concerns over the course of the nineteenth and twentieth centuries. Chapter 6 considers the issue of sexual health, specifically the different responses put in place to deal with sexually transmitted diseases over time and place. Chapter 7 examines the use of psychoactive substances such as alcohol, tobacco and illegal drugs, and considers how the use of these substances came to be seen as problematic. Chapter 8 explores the history of malaria control, a topic with clear relevance to current interventions.

In the final section of the book, we address public health dilemmas of the twentieth century. Chapter 9 examines the development of health systems within welfare states in the West, focusing in particular on the different systems that developed in Germany, Britain and the USA. In Chapter 10, we look at the development of public health in the West in the first half of the twentieth century as it shifted its view away from the environment and towards education and personal responsibility. In Chapter 11, we shift the focus away from the West and turn to international public health, especially the emergence of global health after 1945. Then in Chapter 12 we turn back to the West, to examine the fate of public health in the second half of the twentieth century, and the emergence of new variants of public health, including health promotion. In the final chapter of the book, we consider some of the ways in which history is used in policy and practice.

Each chapter has an overview, learning objectives, a list of key terms, activities, feedback and a brief summary and list of references. Activities are usually based on primary material from the period studied or on later interpretation by historians.

Aim and objectives

The aim of this book is to enable you to employ historical perspectives in the critical evaluation of issues in public health and health services.

After working through the chapters in this book you will be able to:

- Locate developments in public health and health services within historical context, in both the industrialized West and the global South.
- Recognize the nature of historical debate and the contested status of historical claims.
- Analyse original documents so as to be able to assess a significant historical question.
- Evaluate the historical dimensions of ongoing public health issues.

Acknowledgements

This book is the result of collaboration between a group of historians working together at the London School of Hygiene & Tropical Medicine. Virginia Berridge, Martin Gorsky and Alex Mold are responsible for the structure and approach of the book. The chapters were written by a team of authors, and then edited by Alex Mold and

Virginia Berridge. The principal authors of the chapters are as follows: the overview of the book, Virginia Berridge and Alex Mold; Chapter 1, Martin Gorsky, with input from Alex Mold and Virginia Berridge; Chapters 2, 3 and 9, Martin Gorsky; Chapters 4, 6, 10, 12 and 13, Virginia Berridge; Chapters 5 and 11, John Manton; Chapter 7, Alex Mold; Chapter 8, Maureen Malowany and Suzanne Taylor.

In addition, the authors would like to thank Nadja van Ginneken, Ros Plowman and Nicki Thorogood at the LSHTM, and Rachel Crookes from Open University Press who read the draft chapters and made many helpful suggestions for improvements. We would also like to acknowledge the support of Dominic Forrest, who secured permissions for reproduction.

History in public health: The nature and practice of history

Martin Gorsky, Alex Mold and
Virginia Berridge

Overview

This chapter introduces the book, and aims to familiarize you with historical research and writing. The first section asks: what is history? It discusses how the discipline, and specialization in the history of health and medicine, emerged. Next you will examine how historical research and knowledge differs from that in the natural and other social sciences. You will then explore the basic method of primary and secondary source analysis. The chapter concludes with an exercise in source analysis based on the second cholera pandemic of the nineteenth century.

Learning objectives

After working through this chapter, you will be able to:

- describe the development of the historical discipline
- recognize what is distinctive about historical knowledge and research
- comprehend the nature of primary sources and approaches taken to their analysis
- comprehend the nature of secondary sources and explain why historical inter-pretation is always provisional

Key terms

Aeteology/etiology The study of the causes of disease. This may include predisposing factors, whether environmental or genetic, as well as transmission vectors.

Health system Term originating in the mid twentieth century, usually understood as signifying the provision, financing and regulation of primary, secondary and pre-ventive health services. Note that although apparently descriptive, the expression implies the integration of such services.

History of medicine A sub-discipline of history that emerged in the mid-twentieth century, concerned with medical science, population health and health services in the past.

Primary source An original document or artefact *from* the period that is the subject of study.

Professionalization Process involving extensive training, academic qualifications, autonomy, vocational commitment, recognition by the state and restraint of groups of inferior status.

Secondary source A text containing a narrative and/or analytical history of a period or theme produced *after* the period that is the subject of study.

Introduction

Many of you will have little experience of historical study. Indeed, you may remember history lessons from your schooldays as a parade of supposedly important dates, key events in war and politics, and the deeds of 'great' individuals (usually men). Although we cannot promise that these will be entirely absent from this book, we want to suggest that the history of public health is well worth studying. Not only is it inspiring and intellectually stimulating, but an understanding of how past events have shaped the present can helpfully illuminate contemporary challenges. This does not mean we are going to present you with 'lessons of history' on which we can all agree. For while it is certainly possible to reach consensus on *what* happened in the past, the really important questions about *how* and *why* change occurs are much harder to resolve. Before you begin your studies of public health history, this chapter will introduce you to the nature of historical research and knowledge.

What is history?

You may have a ready answer to this question. In colloquial usage, 'history' is shorthand for 'the past'. We may take it to mean absolutely everything that has happened in human experience, or we may think in terms of the past of our nation, region or city, or we may conceptualize history in terms of our own families, our personal 'roots'. However, the origins of the word 'history' are much narrower: it comes from the Latin *historia*, and means a 'story' or narrative account; in other words, the oral or written record of the past. This is an important distinction: history is not 'all and everything' that has happened before; it is a selective account of past events, crafted and delivered by the historian.

The development of the discipline of history

We can imagine, perhaps romantically, the birth of history in ancient societies where tribal elders preserved the collective memory of their people through oral tradition. But we can only confidently start tracking the development of the discipline through the survival of texts. So in Europe we can firmly trace its establishment in the classical period, when Greek and Roman historians began to separate history from myth, and to discuss cause and effect without simply invoking the gods. Their subjects were largely military and political accounts of the empires of Persia, Athens and Rome. The earliest examples in Europe, from around the seventh century ' -C -, were the 'annals' and 'chronicles' produced in monasteries, listing dates and events in the life of the Church, as well natural disasters, war and politics. Historical writing was also a feature of the European cultural Renaissance from the fifteenth century. Political history remained the dominant subject matter, but now explanation of past events was presented in secular rather than religious terms and writers began to strive for an impartial, critical perspective.

It was in the nineteenth century that the historical discipline became established in the universities, accompanied by discussion of the historian's methods: the discovery and dispassionate analysis of original documents – the 'primary sources' – that hold evidence about the past. It was an age of nationalism and the nation-state in Europe and America, so the study of military history, politics and government remained the chief focus. Some of this work contained assumptions about history as a story of progressive betterment; in other words, that the past was worth studying to understand the evolution of liberal societies and their desirable features, such as parliamentary democracy, constitutional government and religious toleration. In Anglophone writing, this idea of 'history as progress' is dubbed 'Whig history' because its leading nineteenth-century exponent, the politician Thomas Macaulay, belonged to the Whig Party (the predecessor of Britain's Liberal Party).

Exercise 1.1

Despite history steadily gaining academic respectability, people sometimes expressed frustration with its shortcomings.

Read the examples of such criticism below and itemize the authors' concerns about the value and meaning of history.

Quotation 1

'Reading modern history is generally the most tormenting employment a man can have. One is plagued with the actions of a detestable set of men called conquerors, heroes, great generals, and we wade through pages loaded with military details. But when you want to know the progress of agriculture, of commerce, and industry, their effects in different ages on each other, the wealth that resulted, its employment and the manners it produced ... all is blank.'

Arthur Young, 1789 (Young, 1794, p. 255) [Young was an English journalist during the early Industrial Revolution, with particular interests in the transformation in agricultural productivity arising from new techniques.]

Quotation 2

'History is more or less bunk. It's tradition. We don't want tradition. We want to live in the present, and the only history that is worth a tinker's damn is the history we make today.'

Henry Ford, *Chicago Tribune*, 1916 (Batchelor, 1994, p. 1) [Henry Ford was an American car-maker and industrialist.]

Quotation 3

'I'm going to give the people an idea of real history. I'm going to start a museum. We are going to show just what actually happened in years gone by.'

Henry Ford, 1919 (Bryan, 2006, p. 11)

Feedback

Quotation 1

Young is concerned that histories of war and great men are completely unrelated to most people's lives. Why, he wonders, can historians not tell us about the development of the economy, the ways in which trade, manufacturing and investment interact, and the resulting changes to social behaviour ('manners').

Quotation 2

Much misquoted as 'History is bunk', this well-known saying is often taken as the quintessential statement of history's irrelevance. Ford seems to be arguing that history and the past are not important in the present; instead, it is wealth creation that really matters.

Quotation 3

This second statement made by Ford qualifies his earlier view. It turns out that Ford was not against history in itself, he just felt that most of it did not tell us 'what actually happened'. Like Young, his idea of 'real history' was the study of work, industry and ordinary people's lives.

The last hundred years have seen a huge expansion in the range and approach of historical writing, which has met all these concerns and more. The following are some of the main developments:

Economic and social history. This approach to history responded to the manifest changes to Western economies and societies in the nineteenth century. The aim was to understand the transformations of farming and industrial production, the growth of internal and international trade, and new patterns of consumption. A related concern was their impact on ordinary people, viewed through the history of population (including past mortality and fertility trends), urbanization, transport, housing, and experiences like work, education and poverty.

Cultural and intellectual history. This approach explored the role of beliefs and ideas as drivers of change. Instead of attributing agency to 'great men', it focused attention on the systems of thought that motivated people to action.

Marxist history. Karl Marx's ideas influenced a whole school of economic and social history. For him, all human societies were moving at different paces through distinct phases determined by their economic 'mode of production'. The first transition was from agrarian 'feudal' societies of aristocrats and peasants to early capitalist societies with a developing middle class engaged in commerce. Next came mature industrial capitalism, in which two hostile classes, the 'bourgeoisie' and 'proletariat' emerged, and finally (Marx hoped) socialism, when the working class would sweep aside their exploiters.

The 'Annales' school. This was a group of French economic and social historians who distinguished *histoire événementielle* (the history of events) from *la longue durée* (long-term change). They believed that before you could make sense of short-term events you needed to study the deep, long-term structures that shaped people's lives, particularly the geographical environment, climate, food and drink, patterns of marriage and fertility, and disease ecology. They also argued that the historian's job was to investigate *mentalité*, to understand and inhabit the very different mental world of people in the past.

Women's history. Although there had been a small number of women in the profession, it was not until the resurgence of feminism in the 1970s that women historians threw down a major challenge. Why was it that half the population was virtually invisible in the '*his*-stories' that had been written until then? Their first aim was to recover the experience of women from the patriarchal neglect of earlier historians, but their impact soon grew as they started to investigate the nature of 'gender'. Masculinity and femininity, they argued, were not essential characteristics, but were learnt and constructed.

Post-colonial history. Scholars from the newly independent nations set out to reclaim and write their own history. An early example was Eric Williams' *Capitalism and Slavery* (1944), in which he argued that far from the slave trade being abolished thanks to enlightened European campaigners, it had ended only because it was no longer economically viable.

History of medicine arrives

The first histories of medicine took a 'Whiggish' approach, whereby scientific advances of Western biomedicine were celebrated as progressive betterment (indeed, some still do). Typically, the form was a description of great doctors of the past and their breakthrough discoveries, and often the authors were doctors themselves.

In mid-twentieth-century America, the history of medicine emerged as an academic discipline in its own right. A key figure was Henry Sigerist, a Swiss national who led the first major department, at Johns Hopkins University, and founded the journal now called the *Bulletin of the History of Medicine* in 1933. Another pioneer was George Rosen, a New Yorker trained in medicine, sociology and public health, whose *A History of Public Health* (1958) was the first attempt to write a survey from earliest times to the present.

In Britain, the specialty emerged in part from interest by public health professionals and was given financial support by the Wellcome Trust, established by the will of the pharmaceuticals magnate Sir Henry Wellcome (d. 1936) to fund both research in medicine and its history. Research units funded by Wellcome bolstered established areas like the history of medical science and health services, but also emerging themes, ranging from professionalization to the cultural history of the body, to colonial and post-colonial medicine.

The nature of historical knowledge

How is history done, and how does it compare with findings in other disciplines?

Why is historical research different?

Readers with a background in the natural sciences should start by considering how historical research differs from that in fields like physics or microbiology. In these areas, to advance knowledge researchers apply a scientific method, proceeding from hypothesis formation to laboratory experiment, to hypothesis refinement, and then repetition of the experiment until the thesis is verified or falsified. The goal is to arrive at laws about the natural world, which not only tell us how things currently behave, but how they will behave in the future.

History is concerned with human behaviour, so we cannot apply this method. All historical events are unique, and because they are unrepeatable, explanatory hypotheses can never be definitively verified or falsified. History, therefore, cannot produce laws about human behaviour, and it cannot be predictive. In a literal sense, there can be no 'lessons' of history.

History is also different from other social sciences that deal with human behaviour in the present. If researchers want to investigate, say, the effectiveness of a health promotion programme, or the impact on patient satisfaction of a new health technology, they have various options open to them. They can conduct an intervention study or a randomized control trial, and they can use different methods to discover their patients' responses, like surveys, interviews, participant observation or focus group discussions. None of this is possible for the historian. Instead, the first problem for any history project is: What evidence has survived that will help me answer my question? In most cases, the further back in time we go, the thinner the evidence base becomes. The situation is not hopeless, however, because for many subjects plenty of documents will have survived. But the problem is that they will have been produced for some other purpose than to answer our particular research question. So, we cannot design a bespoke research instrument. We always have to look at the past through somebody else's eyes.

Exercise 1.2: Is history an art or a science?

Take a moment to read the two quotations below, and then answer the questions that follow:

'History is distinguished from all other sciences in that it is also an art. History is a science in collecting, finding, penetrating; it is an art because it recreates and portrays that which it has found and recognized. Other sciences are satisfied simply with recording what has been found; history requires the ability to recreate.'

Leopold Von Ranke, *The Theory and Practice of History*, nd. 1830s
in Iggers (ed.) 2011 (p. 8)

'...the difficulties historians face in establishing cause and effect relations in the history of human societies are broadly similar to the difficulties facing astronomers, climatologists, ecologists, evolutionary biologists, geologists and palaeontologists. To varying degrees, each of these fields is plagued by the impossibility of performing replicated, controlled experimental interventions.'

Jared Diamond, *Guns, Germs and Steel: A Short History of Everybody for the Last 13,000 Years*, 1997 (p. 424)

1 How far would Ranke and Diamond agree with the statement 'history is not a science'?
2 Do you agree with the statement 'history is an art, not a science'? Give reasons.

Feedback

1 Ranke and Diamond would probably both disagree with the statement that 'history is not a science', but for different reasons. Ranke suggests that history is similar to science in that it requires the collection of data about the world around us, but it is also an art, as historians must recreate the past. So, for Ranke history is both art and science. Diamond raises different issues about the nature of history. By stating that history shares the same difficulty some science subjects experience in being unable to perform controlled experiments, Diamond is pointing out that both history and some natural sciences face similar challenges in verifying hypotheses.

2 There is no 'right' answer to the question as to whether history is an art or a science, and as Ranke and Diamond suggest, it is possible that history is both art and science.

The partial and imperfect nature of historical evidence does put the historian at a disadvantage compared with researchers in other disciplines. And unlike the natural sciences where objectivity can be verified by replicating an experiment, in historical writing there may be higher risks of subjectivity in the selection or interpretation of data.

However, it is important not to make too much of these differences. Researcher bias and imperfect data collection instruments are features of the other social sciences too. With respect to method, historians can aim for the same rigour as other researchers, developing and testing hypotheses or conceptual models, analysing their evidence accurately and critically, and carefully referencing their findings so that later scholars can validate them. Note that even in the natural sciences all knowledge is ultimately provisional and subject to revision. Consider, for example, how Einstein's insights revolutionized Newtonian physics, or how Darwin's theory of evolution shattered existing thought in biology.

An even more forceful criticism has gathered pace in the last twenty years under the influence of *postmodern* literary criticism and philosophy. Postmodernists such as Keith Jenkins and Alan Munslow argue that as soon as historical facts are marshaled within explanatory narratives they become subject to the devices of literary fiction. Hence the empirical content, which can be verified, always comes packaged within an imaginative exercise containing fictive elements such as judgments, values and metaphors, which cannot be validated (Jenkins and Munslow, 2004, pp. 3-4, 9). The attack mounted on history (and other academic subjects) by postmodernism brings into question the objectivity of historians and the very nature of truth. The result, though, has not been to damage the discipline, which remains vigorous and popular. The result, though, has not been to damage the discipline, which remains vigorous and popular. In response to the dilemmas posed by postmodernist criticism historians still strive to present as accurate a picture of the past as possible, while remaining alert to the ways in which their own subjectivities and opinions influence their research and writing. As Richard Evans, Professor at the University of Cambridge, puts it: the past 'really happened, and we really can, if we are very scrupulous and careful and self-critical, find out how it happened and reach some tenable, although always less than final conclusions about what it all meant' (Evans, 1997, p. 253).

Historical methodologies: Use of original sources

So what are the methods by which historians 'find out how it happened'? We work with two categories of data:

- *Primary sources*: the original material from the period that is the subject of our research, and which provides the evidence we interrogate as we explore a question or test a hypothesis.
- *Secondary sources*: the subsequent literature on our topic of interest that we use to discover existing theories and explanations, to establish what primary material has already been used, and how it was interpreted.

We return later to the use of secondary sources. First, what are the main types of primary sources?

Exercise 1.3: Identifying sources

Imagine that you have been asked to write a history of a recent political development in your country. This could be an event such as an election, the introduction of a new policy initiative or a political scandal.

Write a list of the kinds of sources you could gather together to write this history.

Feedback

You may have come up with some or all of the following types of sources:

- Government papers: including correspondence between ministers and civil servants, policy briefing papers, minutes of meetings, etc.
- Media sources: including newspapers, magazines and learned journals, TV and radio news bulletins, news websites and blogs
- Visual sources: including photographs, films and objects
- Personal papers: including private diaries, letters and emails
- Oral sources: including interviews and discussions with some of the people involved in the event

Although we asked you to think about how you would write a history of a very recent event, historians work in a similar way when approaching the past. Of course, not all sources are available to those who work on the more distant past (such as email and oral history), but historians do use many of these different kinds of primary sources. As you will see, all of these primary sources have benefits and drawbacks.

Primary sources for public health

The range of historical resources spans everything from the patterns of field systems that survive in agricultural landscapes to a private letter from a wife to a husband. However, public health history typically concentrates on certain types of documentary source:

'*Official*' *sources.* These are the records of the national and local governments, which, for at least two hundred years in the West, have played a significant role in health. It was national governments that collected statistical data on mortality and commissioned population censuses. They also published reports and enquiries on such subjects as poverty, urban life, the medical profession, sexual health, and alcohol; these contain useful information drawn, just like today, from expert witnesses. Then there are unpublished records, like minutes of committees and briefing notes by civil servants, which allow us to see how policy was developed. Local and municipal governments were also closely involved in areas such as environmental health, hospital provision and maternity care, and again have left published and unpublished records. Each country organizes its official archives slightly differently, but it is usual to find one major repository holding records of national government, then smaller regional or municipal archive offices with more local contents.

Newspapers, professional journals and books. The other major category is 'unofficial' publications, which survive mostly in libraries. Newspapers are a very old form of media, with early examples (in Britain at least) going back to the 1600s, and these can be mined both for the reporting of events and for editorial opinion. Past medical journals are a major source for the changing understandings of disease aetiologies and therapies, and the development of health systems. Many are now available online such as the *New England Journal of Medicine, The Lancet* and the *British Medical Journal.* Printed books by leading doctors or health policy-makers are another source serving the same purpose. From 1879 onwards, the yearbook *Index Medicus* has listed all new books and journal articles in medicine.

Letters, diaries and personal papers. Occasionally, the private papers of individuals have survived. In the case of key actors like scientists and politicians, these can helpfully reveal their intimate thoughts on a subject, rather than those they presented for public consumption.

Visual artefacts. Sources in this category include cartoons, maps, photographs, film, paintings and posters. In addition to those preserved in galleries or museums, many are increasingly available online: check the 'Image Database' of the National Library of Medicine, or the Wellcome Library's 'Wellcome Images' site.

Oral history. Finally, in addition to documentary sources, the contemporary historian also has the opportunity to speak directly to people who lived through the events being studied. As with the private papers mentioned above, this is a very good way of learning about mentalities and motivations of people in the relatively recent past. No less important is the testimony of 'elites', such as scientists and politicians.

The limitations of primary sources

We noted earlier the historian's fundamental difficulty: the sources that have survived are very rarely those that will directly answer the question being posed. Typically, they will have been produced for some purpose quite different from leaving a record for future generations. This means we must approach them with care and critical awareness. Here are some of the difficulties that historians face:

Their fragmentary nature. Historical research can be like doing a jigsaw puzzle for which vital pieces are missing. Sometimes it can be a matter of chance that determines whether a document survives. In other cases, such as with official papers, choices are made about what to keep and what to destroy, and this process of selection determines the evidence available, and thus the conclusions that may be drawn.

Their unreliability. Before we can decide whether a source is a reliable representation of the past, we need to know why it came into being. When first approaching a new source, begin by analysing its 'provenance' (a term used by art-dealers to mean the history of a painting and its past ownership). Ask yourself, when and where was it produced, what was its purpose, who was it for, and who was responsible for creating it? This is the first step in gauging reliability.

Their partisanship. We also need to think carefully about the perspective and position of the writer, for there are many factors that might bias his or her presentation of the past. These include political beliefs, social class, ethnicity, gender and religion.

Problems of visual sources. Just like written text, it is important to treat images with great caution and not assume that they give us unmediated access to the 'real' past. Paintings aim principally for an aesthetic effect rather than faithful reproduction. Posters tell us something about health messages, but next to nothing about how people responded to such messages.

Problems of oral history. Although oral history is direct interview testimony, again proceed with caution. Memory can deceive, or become rosy with time, and interviewees might mislead, perhaps by parroting received opinion, or by taking the opportunity to settle scores.

It is these problems, and the consequent impossibility of accumulating sufficient direct evidence ever to resolve a historical question, which leaves scope for interpretation. Historical 'truth' is therefore no more than an existing scholarly consensus. However, this does not invalidate historical knowledge. Much factual material is uncontentious, and based on broad agreement between researchers who have corroborated their findings from a range of different sources (i.e. triangulation). Rather, it is the analysis of cause and effect, the historical interpretation and explanation, which is subject to change and revision. Historians who think of themselves as social scientists see this process as one of developing and testing hypotheses that will generate convincing theories, albeit always provisional ones. And as we have seen, those of a literary or postmodernist persuasion see it also as an act of imagination, leading to a narrative that tries to convince through presentational devices. In short, then, history is both a body of knowledge *and* an area of disputed interpretation.

Doing history: Cholera in the early nineteenth century

In this final section, we explore some of these themes through studying and interpreting one *primary* and two *secondary* sources. The subject is one that looms large in the history of public health – the cholera pandemics of the nineteenth century. First, some background.

The world experienced six cholera pandemics between 1817 and 1923. The first (1817–1823) originated in the Indian subcontinent and extended west to Turkey and east to Japan; the second (1829–1851) reached Western Europe and the United States, with severe, high mortality epidemics in 1832 and 1848–1849. Cholera returned in four subsequent pandemics: 1852–1859, 1863–1879, 1881–1896 and 1899–1923.

The symptoms of cholera are acute diarrhoea accompanied by vomiting, resulting in severe dehydration and its sequelae. Early descriptions noted its rapid onset, and that in some cases it could lead to death within a few hours; fatality rates could reach about 50 per cent. In 1854, a key breakthrough was made by John Snow, a London physician who argued that cholera was 'communicated by something which acts directly on the alimentary canal' (discussed in more detail in Chapter 3). The comma-shaped bacterium *Vibrio comma* was isolated by Robert Koch in 1883 and this, together with the work of Snow and others, led gradually to the acceptance of the faecal–oral transmission of cholera. Today, the disease can be successfully treated with intravenous saline fluids, oral rehydration and antibiotics.

Exercise 1.4: Cholera in Bilston

Suppose you had the following general research question: 'How did people in the West understand and respond to the cholera epidemics of the mid nineteenth century?' To answer this question, you might begin by collecting and reviewing sources like the one below, a contemporary account of the 1832 cholera pandemic reaching an industrial town in the English Midlands.

Read the extract below and then answer the questions that follow:

'When the disease was raging at Sunderland, and measures of precaution ordered by the Privy Council [*a government committee*] to be taken, the minister at Bilston convened a meeting of the Inhabitants to take the subject into consideration. It was declared by a Medical Practitioner well acquainted with the Inhabitants generally, that the general health was never better at that time; and that it did not appear necessary to resort to any extraordinary means of precaution; which was the unanimous opinion of those present. From the time of holding the said meeting until the Wake [*a public holiday*], there was nothing indicative of any change in the general health of the Inhabitants of this Township. The Wake commenced and was carried on as in years aforetime.

There were the usual festivities, and processions of the various Clubs and Lodges, with their display of flags bearing inscriptions and mottos creditable to their professions. But alas! there was the usual demoralizing pastime of Bull-baiting [*a popular blood-sport in which a bull was attacked by fighting dogs*] continued — that baneful incentive to drunkenness and disorder, notwithstanding it was well known the Cholera was raging at the same time, at the adjoining parish of Tipton.

On the Friday evening August 3rd ... as a thief in the night, the Cholera made its appearance in three houses apart from each other about three hundred yards, situated on each side of the Brook (and of course the lowest ground) in the most densely populated part of the Town; the three points making a figure the form of a triangle ...

Sunday August 5th. On this day three died; one of which was in Hall Street, near to the House where the child died on the day before.

On the same day a Board of Health was formed; and the dead were now buried on the day they died ...

9th. Deaths three. The weather was very hot and but little wind. The smoke from the chimneys ascended perpendicular. The heat was excessive from eight to twelve o'clock in the evening ...

11th. Eleven deaths occurred this day; one of which was a woman who lived near Price's Furnaces, whose husband was at work the previous night — she died in the morning before his return ... The situation of this house in which this woman died, was near to some low ground, to which place, the water and filth from the street had found its way, and had become stagnant, the usual course into the brook having been choked up by the cinder mount. It is remarkable that up to this time the deaths were chiefly confined to filthy courts and close places. In such places the air would have a tendency to become impure, from the collected filth being pent up therein ...

Fear was a strong auxiliary to the spreading of the disease. One who died this day was a stout, robust man, a Spoon-maker, who on the preceding night had in his conversation, expressed some fear he should catch it and die ...

14th. It is worthy of remark, up to this time, there was not the usual appearance of Flies and Swallows ...

15th. There was a thunder storm the last night, which caused the air to be much cooler and refreshing. The number of deaths this day decreased to twelve; three of which were female inmates of the Workhouse. They had been employed in washing the linen. One hundred and eighty families were relieved on this day with mutton and bread, from the subscription raised amongst the wealthier inhabitants, which were but few, compared with the poor and working classes, great numbers of whom were now, from the unsettled state of trade, unable to procure those substantial articles of food …

21st. The Town Surgeons were now sinking under fatigue, in consequence, several Medical Practitioners arrived from Birmingham. Thirty-nine deaths occurred.

22nd. This day died one of the Town Surgeons, whose attention to the wants of his afflicted neighbours, had been incessant by day and by night …

Sunday 26th. Rain at intervals during the day, and the wind N.W. Divine Service was performed as requested at the Board of Health the day before, but the number of deaths this day was truly appalling, being thirty-five …

Sunday, Sept. 16th. The weather was very fine, the air cool and salubrious. The people were in attendance at Church as usual, their countenances were altered from dejection to a smile …

17th. Very fine. Trade and business resumed their former activity – and thanks were given to God for His great Deliverance.'

Extracts from Joseph Price, *A Brief Narrative of the Events Relative to the Cholera at Bilston in the Year 1832* (Bilston, George Price: 1840)

1 What does the source tell us about society's response to cholera in the 1830s?
2 How did people understand cholera?
3 How might the issues of provenance and partisanship affect the reliability of this source?

Feedback

1 *Responses*. There are references to burying the dead on the day they die, a local Board of Health, to doctors caring for patients, to a subscription organized to provide food for the poor.

2 *Understandings*. This source suggests an array of explanations, which varied from divine intervention to immoral behaviour (such as drinking and bull-baiting), to individual vulnerability due to 'fear', to climatic influences, to touch, to the gathering of large crowds. However, there is empirical observation of environmental risk (stagnant water and filth). In the 1830s, then, people lacked the basic knowledge necessary to manage a frightening disease with a high and rapid case fatality. There is no reference to microbial infection or the faecal/oral route of transmission. John Snow's breakthrough lay in the future, as did the laboratory work of French chemist Louis Pasteur in the 1860s, which led to acceptance of the germ theory.

3 *Reliability*. The source was published eight years after the events, so there may be problems of recall. We are not told anything about the author, but he appears to be a layperson not a doctor. His high level of literacy and the fact that he was able to publish such an account might suggest he was part of the urban elite. Indeed, Joseph Price shared his surname with a local industrialist and publisher, so this is possible. We have no clues about the readership, but as publication was in Bilston, this was probably a local pamphlet read by only a few. We would therefore need to triangulate with other similar publications to assess its representativeness.

Now that we have looked at a primary source on understandings of cholera, let us consider how public health historians have treated this subject.

Exercise 1.5: Cholera in England – historical interpretation in a secondary source

Read the extract below from the historian Sheldon Watts and then answer the questions that follow:

'In facing cholera in their own homeland the British medical community were still at sixes and sevens. There was no agreement as to whether this particular fever-like disease was contagious, or whether it was non-contagious and caused by identifiable predisposing causes [*the idea that some individuals have special susceptibility to a disease due to factors like attitude, habits, diet or behaviour*]. If the new cholera were indeed contagious, medical and administrative logic would require quarantines and cordons sanitaires [*a barrier set up to stop the spread of a disease*]. However, as every Briton knew, since the era of the Continental Blockade imposed by Napoleon, Britain's prosperity had depended on its mercantile fleet and world-wide freedom of trade. Fortunately for Britain's continued commercial well-being, an alternative, non-contagious explanation was at hand.

With the arrival of cholera in Sunderland late in 1831 ... local Durham, Northumberland and Newcastle "coal-owners, coal-merchants and other traders" had warned medical reporters that their claim that the cholera was a new disease, probably contagious, brought in by ship from India was "*a rash, ignorant and erroneous judgement*". Following this tongue-lashing by these influential local employers, a committee of eighteen medical doctors "are said to have delivered their unanimous opinion at a public meeting" that the disease was in fact *not* the Indian epidemic but instead some standard English fever which required no administrative response that would cut off trade and shipping.

Coached by medical doctors who were in turn coached by inter-regional traders and bankers, Government after November 1831 saw cholera as "non-contagious". It was a variant of an English fever which could be expected to target those who were predisposed to it by their immoral living, their neglect of family values, their holding of opinions about political matters, and their heavy drinking ...

Ideologues and incipient liberals, seizing the opportunity provided by the cholera, strove purposefully to smash the moral world of the artisan classes. In the interests of middle-class defined "respectability", sporting events were forever cancelled and working men's drinking establishments were vilified and closed down ...'

(Watts, 1997, abbreviated from pp. 186–200)

1 Identify Watts' main arguments.
2 Assess how Watts' assumptions, values and judgements have shaped his argument. Comment on his style of historical writing.

Feedback

1 Watts argues that medical science was not impartial in its response to cholera, and that dominant ideas about aetiology were shaped by economic interests. Because they might have damaged trade, theories that cholera was contagious were rejected in favour of 'predisposing causes'.

2 Watts assumes that there were networks of influence linking medicine with bankers, industrialists and government. Although not explicitly Marxist, the social framework is one of class conflict, particularly in his discussion of the attack on working-class behaviour. Some of his language – 'tongue-lashing', 'smash' – is unashamedly literary, rather than strict scientific reporting. Other historians might disagree with some or all of his judgements, but Watts makes a powerful argument, with implications for public health professionals today.

Finally, here is another historian looking at the same question, of whether theories of cholera's aetiology were determined by economic interests, who came up with a different interpretation.

Exercise 1.6: Cholera in Europe – a different historical interpretation

Read the extract below from the historian Peter Baldwin and then answer the questions that follow:

'An accumulation of experience snowballed across Europe in a broad movement from east to west; a learning curve was traced, with those further along taking their cue from mistakes committed by the firstlings ... Russia's initial decision in favour of strict quarantinism was at first thought to form the mould for the rest of Europe and, indeed, in the beginning its lead was followed by Austria and Prussia. It soon became clear, however, that the information from here was contradictory at best. Russian medical opinion, as well as the reports sent back by foreign observers, conveyed hopelessly mixed signals.

Even in Britain, it would be misleading to portray commercial interests as uniformly opposed to quarantines. Contagion and quarantines were double-edged issues ... other nations would inflict yet harsher measures if they suspected that Britain was giving vessels clean bills of health despite the presence of sickness. The mercantile interests of certain towns did not oppose quarantine as such, seeking only to limit it and shift its costs to the community at large. In other cases merchants were concerned that cholera did not spread among their workers and supported quarantine regulations.

In Britain as elsewhere, opinion on the nature of cholera and the course of prevention was conflicting ... But as elsewhere, increasing experience with the disease impelled many observers away from contagionism [*belief that disease spread by contact*] and towards a sanitationist [*cleansing the environment*] approach ... Britain too benefited from an advanced placement along the geoepidemiological learning curve. The government clearly had no desire to provoke the sorts of disturbances that had accompanied harshly quarantinist measures to the east.'

(Baldwin, 1999, abbreviated from pp. 84, 97–99, 105–7)

1 Identify Baldwin's main arguments and show how they differ from Watts' reading.
2 Do you think that Baldwin's explanation is more convincing than that of Watts?

Feedback

1 Baldwin agrees with Watts that Britain rejected quarantines and the theory that cholera was contagious. However, instead of emphasizing economic interests and class

politics, he argues that Britain developed its policy based on the experience of nations where cholera had already hit. Both medical opinion and commercial interests were genuinely divided, and ordinary people, not just merchants, disliked quarantines.

2 Baldwin's broader geographical focus may give him a better perspective, and it is possible that his comments about diversity of opinion reflect more extensive reading of the underlying sources. But we cannot be sure from this that he has overturned Watts' interpretation. To form a judgement we would need to compare carefully the primary sources each has used, and weigh these against our own reading of original documents. Perhaps even then we would have to conclude that historians can reasonably reach two equally plausible interpretations of past events.

Summary

In this chapter, you have begun to explore the nature and practice of history. History can be defined as the recorded past, and historians work by subjecting primary sources to a rigorous process of analysis to build up a picture about the past. But the past is not uncontested: its meaning and interpretation are always open to debate. This is due to the partial nature of surviving primary sources and the fact that historians bring their own ideas and prejudices to the research and writing of history. The discipline of history has itself undergone many changes over time, and despite the attacks of postmodernists and others, remains a useful tool for analysis. By working through the rest of this book, you will begin to see how and why the history of public health continues to matter.

References and further reading

Baldwin P (1999) *Contagion and the State in Europe 1830–1930.* Cambridge: Cambridge University Press.

Batchelor R (1994) *Henry Ford, Mass Production, Modernism and Design.* Manchester: Manchester University Press.

Bryan FR (2006) *Henry's Attic: Some Fascinating Gifts to Henry Ford and his Museum.* Detroit, MI: Wayne State University Press.

Diamond J (1997) *Guns, Germs and Steel: A Short History of Everybody for the Past 13,000 Years.* New York: W.W. Norton.

Evans RJ (1997) *In Defence of History.* London: Granta.

Iggers GG (ed.) Leopold Von Ranke, *The Theory and Practice of History,* Abingdon: Routledge, p. 8.

Jenkins K and Munslow A (2004) 'Introduction', in *The Nature of History Reader.* London: Routledge.

Huisman F and Harley Warner J (eds) (2006) *Locating Medical History: The Stories and Their Meanings.* Baltimore, MD: Johns Hopkins University Press.

Marwick A (2001) *The New Nature of History: Knowledge, Evidence, Language.* Basingstoke: Palgrave Macmillan.

Pickstone J (1999) The development and present state of history of medicine in Britain, *Dynamis,* 19: 457–86.

Rosen G (1958) *A History of Public Health.* New York: MD Publications.

Tosh J (2006) *The Pursuit of History: Aims, Methods and New Directions in the Study of Modern History* (4th edn). London: Longman.

Watts S (1997) *Epidemics and History: Disease, Power and Imperialism.* New Haven, CT: Yale University Press.

Williams E (1944) *Capitalism and Slavery.* Chapel Hill, NC: University of North Carolina Press.

Young A (1794) *Travels During the Years 1787, 1788, & 1789.* London: W. Richardson.

LIVERPOOL JOHN MOORES UNIVERSITY
LEARNING SERVICES

SECTION 1

Nineteenth century

Public health in the West since 1800: The context   2

Martin Gorsky

Overview

This chapter begins by exploring some of the changing ways in which the activities and organization of public health in the West have been conceptualized during the last two hundred years. It then sketches the outline history of population health in several nations undergoing early economic development. The overall picture is one of improvement, but this raises questions about how these trends can be best explained and what the role of public health has been. The final section discusses material conditions in fast-growing cities in the West that endangered health and shaped the public health response.

Learning objectives

After working through this chapter, you will be able to:

* recognize that definitions of public health have changed over time in response both to the changing disease environment and to economic, political and intellectual factors
* interpret the main trends in life expectancy in the West, and the principal reasons advanced to explain these trends
* identify the material conditions and epidemiological context of nineteenth-century cities, and draw conclusions about the nature of health risks

Key terms

AIDS (Acquired Immunodeficiency Syndrome) A syndrome of viral origin, accepted since the mid-1980s as being caused by HIV (human immunodeficiency virus), although this is still debated by those who cast doubt on the hypothesis. AIDS manifests as a series of potentially fatal infections as a result of severely reduced immunity due to decreased CD4 T-cell lymphocytes. HIV infection is acquired through sexual intercourse, the use of contaminated syringes and through mother-to-child transmission. It is generally asymptomatic for many years before the manifestation of AIDS.

Demographic transition The proposition that when a country undergoes economic modernization that this is accompanied by a shift from a regime of high mortality (a high incidence of deaths in the population) and fertility (a high rate of births in the female population) to a regime of low mortality and fertility. Thus the outcome of the transition will be greater longevity of the population and smaller family size.

Epidemiologic transition The proposition that when a country undergoes economic modernization this is accompanied by a shift from acute infectious diseases to chronic illnesses among the leading causes of morbidity and mortality.

Health promotion Definition of public health adopted through the World Health Organization and the Ottawa Charter (1986) that stressed a wide definition of determinants of health, including environmental issues and those of social justice and equity, rather than just a focus on health education and individual behaviour change.

Medical Officer of Health Local public health official, medically qualified in the UK and working within local government structures until 1974.

'Quack' Derogatory term used to describe unqualified practitioner by qualified one.

Syphilis Caused by the microscopic bacterium *Treponema pallidum*. Usually enters during intercourse with an incubation period of five days to five weeks. Congenital syphilis is transmitted to the foetus inside the infected mother. Multiplicity of possible symptoms, leading, if untreated, to general paralysis of the insane (a late manifestation of syphilis characterized by mental deterioration, speech defects and progressive paralysis). Sometimes called the 'French pox' or the 'Italian disease'.

Urban penalty The proposition that because cities concentrate poor people exposed to unhealthy environments, they are likely to produce higher levels of morbidity and mortality than rural places.

Vaccination The artificial infection of healthy people to induce immunity.

Introduction

If you think of 'public health' in a general sense as any collective action that alleviates or prevents disease, then you could probably trace its beginnings back to the start of human civilization. The first global survey, Rosen's *A History of Public Health* (1958), actually opened four thousand years ago, with the archaeological remains of Mohenjo Daro. Located in present-day Pakistan, this was one of the earliest urban settlements and contained drainage systems and latrines. In medical thought the conceptualization of disease as a common experience rather than individual affliction can be traced at least to the Ancient Greeks. The writings of Hippocrates from about 400 A-B - contained notions of 'endemic' and 'epidemic' disease, the first denoting sicknesses that were characteristic features of particular locations and the second those that could unexpectedly spread through populations.

Thus any attempt to place a start-point on public health history is bound to be arbitrary. In this book, we focus on its modern history, by which we mean the nineteenth and twentieth centuries. The key features of modernity were a transformation in social organization and economic activity, from societies dominated by small, stable populations, living in rural areas or modestly sized towns and engaged in farming or craft production, to those with large numbers of increasingly urbanized people, occupied in the industrial or service sectors. For many of today's high-income nations, this was a process with roots in the eighteenth century that accelerated in the nineteenth. Meanwhile, many currently low- and middle-income countries experienced this period as one of colonization by the West, accompanied by some economic development, only embarking fully on modernization in the mid twentieth century when the imperial era drew to a close (discussed in more detail in Chapter 5 and Chapter 11). Many of the activities, ideas, legal powers and administrative structures that we now associate with public health are best understood as products of this transformation. This chapter will focus on the experience of various Western nations, drawing in particular on examples from Britain, Germany and the United States.

There have been significant changes to the way in which public health has been understood, and the priorities that its practitioners have adopted. We begin, therefore, with some consideration of how public health has been defined and why its meaning has fluctuated.

Exercise 2.1: Conceptualizing public health in modern history – changing definitions from the British past

When did they say it? Read the definitions of public health given below, each of which comes from a different time during the last two hundred years.

For each of them, say which year do you think matches each definition, and explain why. The choices are: 1842, 1903, 1932, 1952, 1976 and 2004.

1 'An examination of the statistics … indicates four main groups of health problems today: those concerned with the ageing of the population, with an unhealthy life style, with mental health and with environmental hazards. Much of the responsibility for ensuring his own good health lies with the individual.'
2 'The primary and most important measures within the province of public administration are drainage, the removal of all refuse of habitations, streets and roads, and the improvement of all supplies of water.'
3 On health visitors: 'I believe in this new departure of carrying sanitation into the home we have not only an important, but almost the only means of further improving the health of the people.'
4 'The science and art of preventing disease, prolonging life and promoting health through the organised efforts and informed choices of society, organisations, public and private, communities and individuals.'
5 'The interpreter of Preventive Medicine uses bacteriology as an aid to diagnosis, prognosis and treatment. He appreciates the processes of infection and swabs throat and nose.'
6 'Preventive medicine … is merely another way of saying health by collective action.'

Feedback

When did they say it?

Definition 1: 1976. This statement is from the booklet *Prevention and Health – Everybody's Business.* Produced by the UK Department of Health and Social Security, it was intended to provoke discussion about the health strategies of the future. Chronic and lifestyle-related diseases were becoming more significant. In place of the old reliance on preventive controls and health services supplied by the state, the policy emphasis was moving to individual responsibility.

Definition 2: 1842. This statement is by Edwin Chadwick, a civil servant and author of a major survey of the people's health in Victorian Britain (Chadwick, 1842; see Chapter 3). Although he wrote before the germ theory of disease causation was advanced, Chadwick believed public health should be synonymous with environmental controls. Sewers, drains, waste collection and fresh water were the priorities.

Definition 3: 1903. This statement is by Alfred Bostock Hill, Medical Officer of Health for Warwickshire (Dingwall et al., 1988, p. 187). Hill was an early specialist in public health in Britain, and his focus was on health behaviours of the individual. Here he argues that with environmental controls now in place, public health improvement hinged on health visitors educating people, particularly working-class mothers, in their own homes.

Definition 4: 2004. This statement is by Derek Wanless, a senior businessman and adviser to the British Treasury, in his report to the government, *Securing Good Health for the Whole Population* (2004). In this twenty-first-century definition, public health is no longer just the concern of government 'experts' and individuals, but a matter for the private sector and local communities, for example working through voluntary sector organizations.

Definition 5: 1932. This statement is by George Newman, then England's Chief Medical Officer, in his book *The Rise of Preventive Medicine* (1932). Writing when the science of bacteriology had become firmly established, he believed that skills and knowledge in this area were now essential for public health doctors. The infections that he had in mind included pulmonary tuberculosis, scarlet fever, diphtheria, syphilis and diarrhoeal diseases.

Definition 6: 1952. This statement is from *In Place of Fear* (1952), a book by Aneurin Bevan, Minister of Health in Britain between 1945 and 1951. Bevan is credited with the creation in 1948 of Britain's National Health Service (NHS), a health system designed to be comprehensive, universal and free at the point of use. In Bevan's view, once the state had guaranteed access to curative health services, then much of the need for public health medicine would disappear.

Though drawn from Britain, these statements give more general hints about how public health in the West has developed over time, whether in response to economic change, to the disease environment, to scientific knowledge or to the political context. Here is a summary:

Broadly, modern public health began in the eighteenth century with efforts by city governments to deal with environmental problems, such as ensuring fresh water supplies, air quality, the removal of waste, and even the location of burial grounds. These efforts intensified in the nineteenth century, when rapid economic growth and mass urbanization coincided with high mortality from infectious diseases such as cholera and typhus. The result was a new body of law and administrative practices that focused on managing the environment to lessen the risk of disease. In its early days, then, public health was more the realm of engineers and politicians than of doctors and epidemiologists. The increasing 'medicalization' of public health followed the scientific breakthroughs of the 1860s, when the French chemist Louis Pasteur formulated germ theory. Bacteriology opened up many new possibilities, for vaccines and pharma-cotherapies, for disease surveillance and screening, and for investigating the safety of food and water. It also prompted interest in health behaviours such as domestic hygiene and safe infant-feeding practices: health education had begun. Thus by the early twentieth century, the concern of public health was moving away from the collective management of the environment to interventions targeted at individuals in the home (see Chapter 10).

By the mid twentieth century, this established focus of public health was beginning to seem less relevant. Insurance- or tax-based systems had extended access to health services and mortality rates had fallen as the old killer diseases like tuberculosis all but disappeared. Meanwhile, economic prosperity and the coming of welfare states had given more people social security and decent housing, and technology had made urban environments safer and more comfortable. In the post-war period, therefore, public health went through a period of reorientation, before finding a new role in addressing the 'diseases of civilization' (see Chapter 12). Cancers and cardiovascular diseases now loomed large in national mortality profiles, and experts increasingly linked these to the lifestyles of modern consumer societies. By the 1990s, however, it had become clear that alongside the new goal of health promotion, the old concern with prevention was still necessary. HIV/AIDS was a reminder to the West that infectious disease risk had not been conquered, while growing evidence of the health effects of climate change put environment firmly back on the public health agenda.

This chapter and the next will cover the nineteenth-century emergence of public health, emphasizing in particular the context of the industrial city. Later in the book (in Chapters 10 and 12), we deal with the subsequent developments, and take the story up to the present day. As a first step, though, we wish to consider the changing picture of population health in the West, against which all this activity took place.

Patterns of population health

Before addressing the actions of governments, doctors and scientists in the cause of public health, we should consider the bodies and pathogens that were their concern. What were the disease regimes in which people lived, and how did these change over the period 1800–2010? To answer this question we need to begin with a brief consideration of demographic history: the study of past population health.

The 'gold standard' method for measuring population health is the examination of patterns of mortality. The reason for this is that since the eighteenth century it became increasingly common for nation-states to compel citizens to register births, marriages and deaths. Thus we have (in theory at least) a comprehensive and universal record of deaths to analyse. Moreover, death is a robust indicator. Unlike sickness, which was only occasionally recorded and is highly subjective, death is a state that can be objectively defined and measured. Therefore, we can calculate trends over time from these data, like changing life expectancy, mortality rates (the proportion of deaths per population living) and the profile of fatal diseases.

Table 2.1 shows mean life expectancy at birth in a selection of industrialized nations. The year in which each series starts reflects the year in which national statistics became available for the different countries. Typically, vital events like birth and death were recorded either by religious or civil officials, and although there are plenty of gaps in the earliest records, scholars believe that these data do give us an accurate picture of trends over time.

Table 2.1 Life expectancy (years) in several Western countries, 1750–1993

Country	1750–1759	1800–1809	1850–1859	1880	1900	1930	1950	1993
England	36.9	37.3	40.0	43.3	48.2	60.8	69.2	76.2
France	27.9	33.9	39.8	42.1	47.4	56.7	66.5	77.4
Sweden	37.3	36.5	43.3	48.5	54.0	63.3	71.3	78.1
Germany	—	—	—	37.9	44.4	61.3	66.6	76.2
Italy	—	—	—	35.4	42.8	54.9	65.5	77.7
Netherlands	—	32.2	36.8	41.7	49.9	64.6	71.8	77.0
USSR	—	—	—	27.7	32.4	42.9	64.0	65.4
USA (white population)	—	—	41.7	47.2	50.8	61.7	69.4	75.7
Australia	—	—	—	49.0	55.0	65.3	69.6	77.9
Japan	—	—	—	35.1	37.7	45.9	59.1	79.4

Source: Modified from Livi-Bacci (2001, p. 97).

Exercise 2.2: Understanding the 'health transition' – trends in life expectancy

What would you highlight as the main patterns in Table 2.1?

Feedback

The figures tell a very simple story: from a rather uncertain start in the late eighteenth century health in the developed world, as measured by length of life, has improved dramatically. In the 1850s, mean life expectancy for a white American was about 42 years, and by 1993 about 76 years. You can see similar patterns in Western Europe and Japan.

You might also have noticed some intriguing trends within this over-arching picture. The absence of early data on non-white Americans (i.e. minorities like native Americans or African slaves and their descendants) reminds us that historical statistics are not neutral, but reflect the political inequalities of the time in which they were collected. Also note Japan's trajectory, with a slow start followed by major gains since the 1950s, before it overtook Sweden as best performer from 1978. In part, this reflects Japan's post-war economic miracle, but growing prosperity does not explain everything; commentators also point to factors like its more egalitarian distribution of wealth, the benign low-calorie diets favoured by its people, and their willingness to respond to public health campaigns.

Now consider Figure 2.1, which presents annual time series data for a single country, England, over a very long period. This will allow you to home in on the trend over time in more detail, allowing you to pose questions about causal factors.

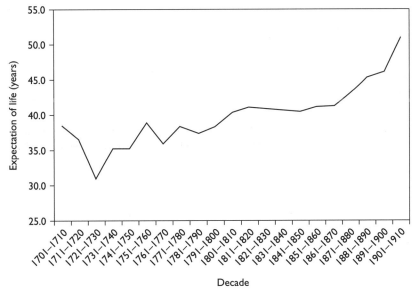

Figure 2.1 Life expectancy in England, 1701–1910

Source: Harris (2004, p. 114)

There are two things you need to know to help you read this graph. First, England is often described as the first nation to experience an 'Industrial Revolution'. This term may conjure up images of factory production, textile manufacturing, engineering, mining and so on, but it meant much more besides, like a powerful service sector, surging agricultural productivity and rapid urbanization. Although the timing of English economic 'take-off' is hotly debated, indicators like booming textiles output typically trace this to the mid eighteenth century. The exact point at which industrialization began to feed through into greater individual prosperity is also debatable, although there is no doubt that it did: one estimate of real per capita expenditure on consumption suggests a rise from £9.3 in the 1770s to £14.6 in the 1820s, to £22.9 in the 1850s (Crafts, 1985, p. 94).

Second, data gathering on births, marriages and deaths in England was not mandatory before civil registration began in 1837. This means that the trend shown in the first part of the graph is not based on systematically collected national statistics, but on a sample of church records. In fact, it resulted from a truly massive research project, in which historians scoured England's parish churches, collecting all the surviving registers they could find. They ended up with 404 registers, from about 10,000 parishes overall, and they then analysed the data, presenting the results as a proxy for the national experience (Wrigley and Schofield, 1989).

Exercise 2.3: Understanding the 'health transition' – the trend for life expectancy in a national case study

With the above two points in mind:

1 Describe the main trends of Figure 2.1.
2 Provide an explanation for your observations.

Feedback

1 As in Table 2.1, there is one overarching story told by the graph in Figure 2.1, of rising life expectancy and thus of a long-term improvement in population health. From a low point of around 31 years in the 1720s, the mean lifespan increased to about 50 years by the early twentieth century. The timing of the rise coincides fairly closely with what is known about England's transition to an industrial economy. Indeed, here is one of the earliest examples of the now familiar relationship between development and health improvement.

2 You may also have speculated about some of the trends over shorter periods, because clearly there was not an unbroken sequential rise. First, note that only from 1800 onwards is the trend line smooth, while in the eighteenth century there were some striking oscillations in the rate. What might account for this? One possibility is that it is an artefact of the underlying data, and that the more sparse availability of the parish registers further back in time has undermined accuracy. However, the historians responsible, Wrigley and Schofield, have staunchly defended their method; they verified their results by plotting death rates from the parish registers for the post-1837 period too, and showed these were close enough to the civil registration data to be reliable. So, based on the assumption that these were real trends, you might have speculated that the causes were war, famine or epidemic diseases.

Historians who have worked on this problem explain the eighteenth-century pattern in terms of the disease environment and food supply. The temporary trough in the late 1710s seems to have been related to hot, dry summers and mortality peaks of typhoid and dysentery. These were followed by a succession of poor harvest years in the 1720s, which are thought to have weakened nutritional status and left people susceptible to endemic and epidemic diseases. In the absence of comprehensive medical certification of deaths the true cause is not known, but contemporary accounts mention smallpox, typhus and influenza. Records from the 1780s refer to particularly intense epidemic 'fever' (typhus).

Perhaps the most puzzling aspect of the graph is that after trending upwards between the 1790s and 1820s, when industrialization was in full swing, mean life expectation then hit a plateau with no further improvement until the 1870s. If there were a straightforward relationship between economic growth, rising individual prosperity and improving health status, this is not what one would expect. Perhaps the answer is that the relationship was *not* straightforward. The most plausible explanation of the temporary hiatus in the long upward trend relates to living conditions. One of the contradictions of development was that standards of living rose unevenly across different groups in the population. British industrialization was characterized by rapid urban growth, in which a comparatively low-skilled and low-waged labour force crowded into unhealthy town environments that exacted an 'urban penalty' of heightened mortality. As we will see, it was largely in response to the risks of urban living that modern public health emerged.

Before considering these urban environments in more detail, let us add a final piece of the jigsaw. We know that life expectation was increasing, and that epidemic and nutrition crises were receding, but exactly which diseases were being 'conquered'? What were the great killers of the nineteenth century, and how did the disease profile change in the twentieth century?

Table 2.2 breaks down the life expectancy gains since the late nineteenth century by cause of death in two case-study countries, England and Italy. Once again the source is mortality registration records, which in England, for example, had to be certified by a doctor when specifying the cause of death. As before, we need to acknowledge problems in the accuracy of certification. This is not surprising, as the classification of diseases is constantly evolving as knowledge improves. In the nineteenth century, for example, diphtheria and scarlet fever were not fully distinguished until 1868, typhus and typhoid until 1869. Even today the issue of co-morbidities complicates correct registration, and discord between post-mortem and certification verdicts demonstrates the difficulties of the practice. Despite all that, the sheer number of observations from which these figures are constructed should give us a reasonably consistent picture.

Table 2.2 Life expectancy gains in England (1871–1951) and Italy (1881–1951) by contributing causes of death

Cause of death	England Gains in e_0 (years)	(%)	Italy Gains in e_0 (years)	(%)
Infectious diseases	11.8	42.9	12.7	40.1
Bronchitis, pneumonia, influenza	3.6	13.1	4.7	14.8
Disease of the circulatory system	0.6	2.2	0.8	2.5
Diarrhoea and enteritis	2.0	7.3	3.4	10.5
Diseases of infancy	1.8	6.5	2.3	7.3
Accidents	0.7	2.5	0.5	1.6
Tumours	−0.8	−2.9	−0.4	−1.3
Other diseases	7.8	28.4	7.7	24.3
Total	27.5	100.0	31.7	100.0

Source: Modified from Livi-Bacci (2001, p. 98). e_0 = life expectancy at birth.

Exercise 2.4: Understanding the 'health transition' – life expectancy and cause of death

What are main messages of Table 2.2?

Feedback

Table 2.2 shows that almost two-thirds of the gain in life expectancy was due to the declining mortality from 'infectious diseases' (e.g. measles, scarlet fever, diphtheria), and from other communicable diseases: respiratory illnesses like bronchitis and influenza and intestinal diseases like diarrhoea and enteritis.

Breaking down the life expectancy gains by age, it is clear that the decline in infant and childhood mortality (under 15 years) in particular underlie the decline in mortality. Two hundred years ago death was more common at all ages, especially for infants and young children, and for young adults too. By the late twentieth century, death was increasingly confined to the latter part of the life cycle: to old age.

To sum up so far, this shift in mortality patterns was an element of what is often called the *demographic transition*. The argument is that with economic modernization societies moved from regimes of high mortality and fertility to regimes of falling death and birth rates. In the case of much of the West, this meant a rise in life expectancy at birth from 34–37 years to 75–79 years by the late twentieth century, and a shift to smaller families – in England, for example, from a fertility rate of five to six children per woman to one to two.

This lengthening of life, decline in infant mortality and increase in the chance of survival to old age is sometimes dubbed the *health transition*. We need to be cautious about this term, because increased longevity does not necessarily mean people lived more healthy lives. Morbidity data are fragmentary, and some sickness insurance records suggest that falling mortality meant rising levels of sickness, particularly among older people. Nonetheless, the overall change is clear. Finally, the health transition was underpinned by what the scholar Abdel Omran called an *epidemiologic transition*. He proposed that development always heralded a shift from an age of 'pestilence and famine' to a period of 'receding pandemics', and finally a phase in which 'pandemics of infection are gradually displaced by degenerative and man-made diseases as the chief form of morbidity and primary cause of death' (Omran, 1971, pp. 536–7).

Again we need to be cautious about assuming these are uniform and inevitable outcomes, for every country and region will display its own characteristics. Nonetheless, population history suggests that a health transition in the developed world has been the feature of the period we are going to study. But how do we explain this? What might the causal relationship have been between economic modernization and health improvement?

Exercise 2.5: Explaining the health transition

List in order of importance some factors that you would hypothesize were the causes of the rise in life expectancy in the West since the eighteenth century. You should draw on your own understanding of the factors underlying health improvement, perhaps in a low-income country today.

Feedback

You might have attributed the greatest importance to advancements in medical science and the new cures that followed. Or you might have stressed the growth of health services and the capacity of public health strategies to curb infectious disease.

Alternatively, you might have considered reasons why rising individual prosperity might have benefited health, such as the better diets and housing that could be purchased.

It might surprise you to learn that no definitive explanation of the historical rise in life expectancy has been arrived at. In Chapter 13, we examine in more detail the debates surrounding this question when we focus on the McKeown thesis. However, six major factors have been identified as crucial, even if historians are not yet in a position to assign relative importance to them. They are as follows:

1 *Medicine.* The period saw the emergence of what we now term 'biomedicine', an understanding of health and disease based on the natural sciences such as chemistry, biology, physiology and anatomy. During the nineteenth century, a scientifically trained medical profession emerged, recognized by governments as distinct from 'quack' practitioners. In addition to Pasteur's germ theory, medical science produced new therapies, including the smallpox vaccine, the application to surgery of anaesthesia, antisepsis and transfusion, and the diphtheria antitoxin. In the twentieth century, there followed the BCG vaccine for tuberculosis, the sulphonamides, penicillin (antibiotics) and chlorpromazine (the anti-psychotic drug). There was also tremendous growth in the provision of health workers, and institutions such as hospitals, clinics and health centres, through which biomedical practitioners and therapies could be accessed.

2 *Levels of wealth.* Comparisons between countries leave no doubt that there was a close correlation between gross national product (GNP) and life expectancy during the transition in the West (GNP is a standard indicator of levels of output and hence relative economic development). However, this was not a direct and consistent relationship – comparative cross-national rankings of health indicators could differ from rankings of wealth. As we noted in the case of Britain, we need to know more about how wealth was distributed and how living conditions changed to understand the relationship.

3 *Nutritional status.* The most probable reason why rising wealth meant better health is that people enjoyed superior diets. As the quantity and quality of food available to populations improved, so did nutritional status, and thus the body's capacity to resist disease.

4 *Public health programmes.* In addition to individualized medicine and private consumption, the period also saw a number of public health interventions. In the nineteenth century, key activities were the building of sewerage and fresh water systems, but they also included mandatory smallpox vaccination, the appointment of public health doctors and the establishment of isolation hospitals. Rising wealth made these initiatives possible, but political choices mattered too.

5 *Individual behaviour.* Whatever the experts may say, it is individuals who determine their own health practices. Behaviour changed in areas such as domestic hygiene, with the use of soap and laundering of clothes, in sexual relations, with the adoption of contraceptive practices, and in the consumption of food and milk, with attention to diets and to safe infant feeding.

6 *Education.* Related to these developments was the spread of education and literacy, which allowed people to become better informed of new knowledge about bacteria and infection, and thus perhaps to modify behaviour. The schooling of women, hitherto more often excluded than men, was particularly important in this regard.

Although the six causes listed above relate to human agency, some factors may have been outside human control. There is evidence that the virulence of diseases can rise and fall autonomously, and in the nineteenth/twentieth centuries, smallpox, scarlet fever and the streptococcal infections that cause puerperal fever have been cited as examples of where this may have been a contributing factor.

Health and the city

So far, we have suggested that public health in its modern form arose in response to the environmental problems of the nineteenth-century city. We have also seen that this was a period of sustained economic development, which over the long run brought major improvements in health. However, it was an uneven process, with mortality risk from some infectious diseases remaining stubbornly high. The remainder of this chapter brings into view the 'urban penalty' to which public health responded, and we draw on the experience of England, Germany and the United States as examples.

The pace of urbanization

The first point to grasp is just how rapid the rise was in population and urbanization that accompanied economic growth. Tables 2.3 and 2.4 present some raw statistics that

Table 2.3 Population growth and urbanization

Year	Europe		England and Wales		Germany	
	Population (millions)	Percent urban	Population (millions)	Percent urban	Population (millions)	Percent urban
1600	78	8	4	6	16	4
1700	81	9	5	13	15	5
1750	94	9	6	17	17	5
1800	123	10	9	20	24	5
1850	177	17	18	41	34	17
1890	230	30	29	62	49	28

Note: urban = towns of 10,000 or more.

Table 2.4 The growth of major cities

Birmingham		Hamburg		Chicago	
Year	Population	Year	Population	Year	Population
1700	9 000	1821	180 000	1840	4 470
1750	24 000	1850	200 000	1850	29 963
1800	74 000	1870	300 000	1870	298 977
1850	233 000	1900	750 000	1890	1 099 850
1900	522 182	1913	1 000 000	1910	2 185 283

Sources: de Vries (1984, pp. 36, 47–8); England and Wales Census of Population; Evans (2005); US Census Bureau, Census of Population and Housing.

help us to conceptualize this. Table 2.3 shows Europe's population in millions, and also that of England and Wales and of Germany, along with the proportion of those populations living in large cities. Table 2.4 illustrates the pace of growth in three vast cities. Birmingham, in the English Midlands was an industrial hub of a coal and iron mining region; it specialized in manufacturing metal goods and engineering. Hamburg, on the mouth of the River Elbe in Germany, was Northern Europe's main grain out-port, with an economy based on the docks, shipbuilding, processing and services. Chicago, the metropolis of the American Mid-West, was another transport hub and centre of manufacturing, processing and meat-packing.

Exercise 2.6: Urbanization rates and health

1 What are the main patterns of urbanization shown in Tables 2.3 and 2.4?
2 Suggest some of the possible impacts on health that might arise from these trends.

Feedback

After a gentle expansion in the seventeenth century Europe's population growth accelerated, almost trebling in size between 1700 and 1890. The pace of change was faster and earlier in England, but later in Germany where industrialization intensified in the late nineteenth century. England was distinguished by an unprecedented degree of urbanization, with two-thirds of its people in large cities by the 1890s. Change was even more rapid in major industrial cities like Birmingham, which grew seven-fold between 1800 and 1900, Hamburg, which grew five-fold between 1850 and 1913, or Chicago, whose growth rate was even more striking.

Unless carefully planned and governed, rapid development meant that infrastructure did not keep pace with population demand. If this led to poor housing, or insufficient amenities like refuse disposal or fresh water, then health might be at risk. Poverty and overcrowding might exacerbate these risks, so that epidemic diseases could lead to periodic crises.

Health risks in the industrial city

Empirical detail needs to be added to these speculations. Here are some key points based on historical studies of urban conditions:

Occupational health. Before health and safety regulation or workers' compensation laws, industrial labour could carry serious health risks. For example, a British survey in 1897 that took the mortality rates of agricultural workers as its baseline (100) found that those of urban workers, such as cutlery and scissor makers (407) and pottery and earthenware workers (453), were far higher.

Housing. There was almost no public housing in the nineteenth century, although philanthropy provided a small amount. National and municipal governments slowly began to take on slum clearance powers, although this did not always help the poor. For instance, Baron Haussmann's project of building the 'grands boulevards' in Paris, 1850–1870, actually decreased available accommodation for the working class. Thus housing was mostly unplanned and left to the market, where quality might be jeopardized by the profit motive.

Overcrowding. One result was severe overcrowding. New York was the world leader in population density: in 1894, when skyscrapers were in their infancy, there were 986 people per acre in lower Manhattan, including one five-block area with 300,000 inhabitants. The 1901 census for Glasgow, Scotland, recorded 'persons per room' in the city, and calculations showed that where families lived in three-room accommodation mortality rates stood at 13.7, but where whole families lived in a single room they were 32.7. Thus it is likely that overcrowding mattered, especially during epidemics of diseases transmitted through aerial or faecal/oral routes.

Sewerage. Toilets, or 'privies', were rarely private amenities, but typically shared between houses. In London in the 1880s, for example, the ratio was 40 inhabitants to one privy. There were three common forms: the wooden 'vault privy', built over a pit, or 'midden', which was regularly emptied by 'scavengers'; the 'pail privy', where excreta fell into a large bucket, also used to hold ash from household fires; and the flushing 'water-closet' made of porcelain and plumbed into urban water and main drainage systems. In Birmingham in 1875 there were 35,000 vault privies, 7000 pail privies, and only 8000 of the more hygienic water closets (recall Birmingham's population size). Thus people might defecate into pots at home and throw the refuse into watercourses, outdoor dung heaps and cesspools, or street drains intended for carrying rainwater. Early attempts to solve the problem could backfire, as in Hamburg where an untreated sewage outflow into the Elbe was so close to the harbour that the tide often failed to wash it away.

Refuse. Related to sewerage was the general problem of 'nuisances' (i.e. rubbish, garbage) collected in heaps on the street. This was an era of horse-drawn transport, and in Brooklyn, for example, 200 tons of horse manure was left on the roads each day. Organic food waste was the other major element (New Yorkers apparently consumed 750,000 watermelons per annum around 1900) along with ash from coal fires. Refuse heaps could be breeding grounds for pests and insects with concomitant health risks ranging from skin problems to typhus and diarrhoeal diseases.

Fresh water. Access to clean water for bathing, laundry, cooking and drinking was poor. Most houses did not have piped water: in the 1840s only one in five dwellings in Birmingham had mains water, and even in 1904 there was one tap per fourteen houses on average in parts of Manchester. Many cities allowed private contractors to supply water from standpipes for a fee in poor neighbourhoods, but the cost and inconvenience limited consumption. In 1859, it cost one penny for three buckets in Burton on Trent, and a typical working-class family would spend three pennies per week for all their washing and cooking. Early municipal waterworks could exacerbate problems if water was drawn unfiltered from rivers or lakes polluted with sewerage or industrial waste. Chicago opened its first waterworks in 1840, drawing fresh water from 600 feet from Lake Michigan, but as sewerage entering the lake increased it moved the source pipe, in 1866, two miles out from the shoreline. By the late nineteenth century, technologies of sand filtration and chlorination led to greater safety, although cities still needed to find the necessary combination of investment capital and political will to implement these solutions (Melosi, 2000, pp. 79–81; Wohl, 1983, pp. 62–3, 98, 282, 289; Evans, 1987, p. 140).

To consolidate some of these ideas, let us turn to two visual sources. Figure 2.2 shows the street plan of a slum area in the city of Nottingham in 1844; this was a typical industrial city in the English Midlands whose economy was centred round textile production, especially the famous Nottingham lace. Figure 2.3 is a photograph from 1890 of vault privies in Hamburg's working-class Alley Quarter.

Exercise 2.7: Visual sources for health risks in the industrial city

Comment on the images in Figures 2.2 and 2.3 from a public health perspective.

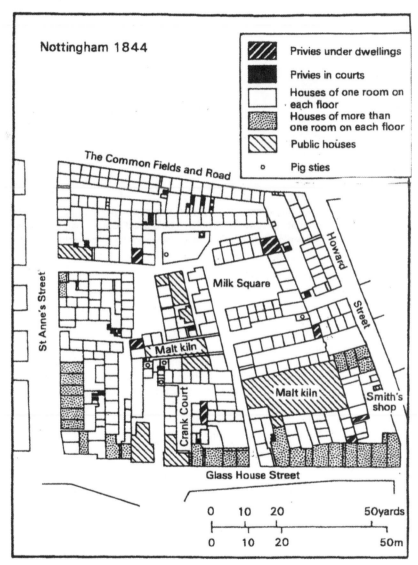

Figure 2.2 Street plan of an area of Nottingham, 1844

Source: Langton and Morris (1986, p. 174)

Feedback

Figure 2.2 shows a working-class area of Nottingham in which the only substantial houses, with more than one room per floor, are those fronting onto the main streets;

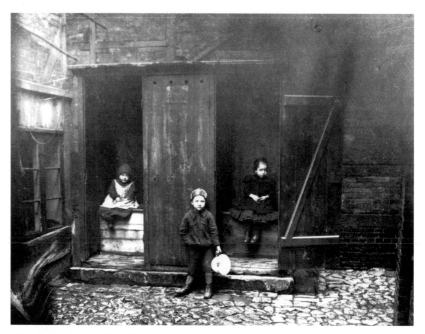

Figure 2.3 Vault privies in Hamburg's Alley Quarter

Source: Evans (2005; original in Staatliche Landesbildstelle Hamburg)

possibly these are older dwellings on whose adjoining land subsequent development took place. Most houses are small and limited to one room per floor, suggesting construction aimed at meeting demand for cheap, tightly packed accommodation. Unlike twentieth-century developments, where street layout is often light, spacious and on a grid system, here the roadways are alleys opening onto a series of small squares, or 'courts'. Most houses do not have their own adjacent privy, and these are shared between many households and typically located under buildings or in courts. Some households keep pigs, and this is suggestive of food refuse heaps in the open spaces. Two industrial buildings, malt kilns for brewing beer, are seen to abut housing. The only social amenities visible are the public houses, where beer is served. Your comments therefore probably centred on the health risks of overcrowded city dwellings with unhygienic sewerage, an environment conducive to the spread of some infectious diseases.

Figure 2.3 shows vault privies with wooden seats that lack a water flushing mechanism, so it is therefore hard to maintain cleanliness. This, coupled with shared use by multiple households, suggests they may have been sites of heightened risk from diseases of faecal-oral transmission, such as typhoid, other enteric diseases and, in epidemic years, cholera. Finally, you may have wondered if the photo was posed for advocacy purposes, and indeed Hamburg voluntary associations were then campaigning for sanitary reform.

Readers based in low-income countries may have seen for themselves the health effects of explosive urban growth. If so, you may be wondering how nineteenth-century epidemiologists and public health doctors responded to what they saw. We close this chapter with a look through the eyes of some proto-epidemiologists.

Figure 2.4 shows a page from England's *Decennial Supplement of the Registrar of Births Marriages and Deaths*, in which statisticians summarized the annually collated mortality data to produce findings on patterns and trends. They also incorporated variables from the Census of Population taken every ten years. Shown here is the male experience for the city of Wolverhampton. This was a characteristic town of the English Industrial Revolution, situated near Birmingham in the 'Black Country', so called because of the smoke pollution from its coal-mines, forges and metal workshops (nail-making was a specialty).

270   *Causes of Death in the Ten Years 1851–60. — Males.*   [DIV. VI.

Mean Population, 1851–61, and Deaths in Districts during the 10 Years 1851–60.

CAUSES OF DEATH.	ALL AGES.	Total under 1 Year.	1	2	3	4	Total under 5 Years.	5–	10–	15–	20–	25–	35–	45–	55–	65–	75–	85 & upwds.
							379.—WOLVERHAMPTON.											
Mean Popul^n, 1851–61	59163	–	–	–	–	–	8592	6993	6226	5612	5742	9585	7304	4714	2734	1246	365	50
TOTAL DEATHS	16830	5492	2088	1001	554	335	9470	711	351	358	447	869	996	988	1003	929	575	133
Small-pox	250	58	36	32	17	19	162	36	8	8	11	18	3	3	1	–	–	–
Measles	664	106	250	160	73	30	619	40	2	–	2	1	1	–	–	–	–	–
Scarlatina	641	47	118	128	104	78	475	121	30	8	4	1	–	1	1	–	–	–
Diphtheria	53	8	8	7	6	6	35	11	1	3	1	–	1	1	–	–	–	–
Whooping-cough	278	135	77	34	13	9	268	10	–	–	–	–	–	–	–	–	–	–
Typhus	806	68	76	73	55	38	310	116	54	54	48	57	52	55	25	23	10	2
Cholera, Diarrh., Dysent^y	1096	638	209	54	22	2	925	18	5	2	4	16	11	25	32	26	27	5
Other Zymotic Dis.	557	144	78	49	39	31	341	31	11	12	6	24	34	26	30	26	14	2
Cancer	86	3	1	1	–	1	6	–	2	1	3	8	8	9	14	17	18	6
Scrofula, Tabes Mesent.	324	141	70	27	16	8	262	15	4	6	8	8	7	11	1	2	–	–
Phthisis	1341	106	57	34	10	6	213	37	34	94	138	273	267	151	98	30	6	–
Hydrocephalus	179	70	55	21	15	6	167	7	5	–	–	–	–	–	–	–	–	–
Diseases of Brain	2030	1178	133	62	31	14	1418	34	20	27	30	45	75	106	97	117	52	9
Heart Dis. and Dropsy	690	36	22	12	12	4	86	19	18	21	18	48	81	134	133	94	34	4
Dis. of Lungs	3236	1068	544	192	72	33	1909	75	16	23	42	105	172	209	293	271	113	8
Dis. of Stom. and Liver	609	163	34	15	5	4	221	16	12	13	10	33	64	71	98	53	16	2
Dis. of Kidneys	146	–	3	1	2	1	7	8	3	3	6	12	25	21	20	26	10	5
Dis. of Gener. Organs	3	2	1	–	–	–	3	–	–	–	–	–	–	–	–	–	–	–
Diseases of the Joints	38	2	1	–	–	1	4	5	2	–	5	7	6	–	6	1	2	–
Diseases of the Skin	24	7	6	–	1	–	14	1	1	–	–	–	2	1	2	1	2	–
Childbirth and Metria	–	–	–	–	–	–	–	–	–	–	–	–	–	–	–	–	–	–
Violent Deaths	1089	39	41	37	45	37	199	89	115	77	98	191	144	102	41	21	10	2
Other Causes	2690	1473	268	62	16	7	1826	22	8	6	13	22	43	57	108	220	273	92

Figure 2.4 Causes of death among males in the ten years 1851–1860

Note: phthisis = pulmonary tuberculosis

Source: General Register Office (1864)

As you look at the page, put yourself in the place of these early medical statisticians, who were starting with an almost blank page. There was no International Classification of Diseases, so they had to develop their own categories. Statistics was in its infancy, and applied techniques like correlation analysis and significance testing still lay in the future. These were the pioneers, who had to decide what and how to measure.

Exercise 2.8: The early measurement of urban health

Comment on the strengths and weaknesses of the extract from *Decennial Supplement of the Registrar of Births Marriages and Deaths* in analysing population health.

Feedback

Strengths

Clearly, a major effort went into quantifying differential mortality by age, by gender (note that there are also tables for females), by cause and by place. Wolverhampton is recorded as District 379, suggesting that there were plenty of other areas with which comparison might be made. There is a row showing mean population, presumably derived from the census totals, and these could be used to calculate mortality rates according to age, gender, place and cause, which could then form the basis of such comparisons. Spatial comparisons such as this could provide insight into the relationship of health to other crude indicators from a census, such as population density, occupational mix and age structure, or from taxation data, as a proxy for wealth. The age breakdowns are especially useful, with the disaggregated details of the under-5s graphically portraying infant and early childhood mortality. The 'under one year' category indicates the scale of perinatal and neonatal mortality. Indeed, these data show strikingly the extent to which the low mean life expectancy of the time was caused by very high death rates in early years of life. The disease classification is rudimentary but could give some idea of the proportion of deaths from infectious diseases that might have been preventable. Note the high proportion of violent deaths of these men and boys; this probably refers to injuries and accidents in heavy industries, then unprotected by child labour laws or health and safety legislation.

Weaknesses

Probably of most concern to a present-day reader will be the diagnostic categories. Indeed, this is from a period before microbial transmission of disease was understood, and the description 'zymotic' disease refers to understandings of aerial contagion emanating from rotting waste matter, whose movement was thought to be climatically determined. Some problem areas are the unspecific nature of the large categories 'diseases of the lung' and 'diseases of the brain', which caused numerous deaths, and the large number of 'other causes'.

Summary

This chapter has demonstrated that the conceptualization of 'public health' is not fixed but has altered over time in response to changing patterns of disease and to political, economic and intellectual influences. Economic development in the West led to a long-term rise in life expectancy. However, there was a period in the mid nineteenth century when poorer city-dwellers were exceptionally vulnerable to infectious diseases. Weak urban infrastructure was part of the problem. The set of public health practices and organizational structures with which we are familiar emerged in the nineteenth century, and was focused in particular on the environmental impacts on health of the industrial city. This is the theme of Chapter 3.

References and further reading

Bevan A (1952) *In Place of Fear*. London: Heinemann.

Chadwick E (1842/1965) *Report on the Sanitary Condition of the Labouring Population of Great Britain* (edited by MW Flinn). Edinburgh: Edinburgh University Press.

Crafts N (1985) *British Economic Growth during the Industrial Revolution*. Oxford: Clarendon Press.

Department of Health and Social Security (1976) *Prevention and Health – Everybody's Business*. London: HMSO.

de Vries J (1984) *European Urbanization, 1500–1800*. London: Methuen.

Dingwall R, Rafferty A-M, and Webster C (1988) *An Introduction to the Social History of Nursing*. London: Routledge.

Evans RJ (1987) *Death in Hamburg: Society and Politics in the Cholera Years*. London: Penguin.

General Register Office (GRO) (1864) *Supplement to the 25th Annual Report of the Registrar-General of Births, Deaths and Marriages in England and Wales*. London: HMSO.

Harris B (2004) *The Origins of the British Welfare State*. Basingstoke: Palgrave Macmillan.

Kirk D (1996) The demographic transition, *Population Studies*, 50 (3): 361–87.

Langton J and Morris RJ (eds) (1986) *Atlas of Industrializing Britain, 1780–1914*. London: Methuen.

Livi-Bacci M (2001) *A Concise History of World Population* (3rd edn). Oxford: Blackwell.

Melosi M (2000) *The Sanitary City: Urban Infrastructure in America from Colonial Times to the Present*. Baltimore, MD: Johns Hopkins University Press.

Newman G (1932) *The Rise of Preventive Medicine*. London: Oxford University Press.

Omran A (1971) The epidemiologic transition: A theory of the epidemiology of population change, *Milbank Memorial Fund Quarterly*, 29: 509–38.

Porter D (1999) *Health, Civilization and the State*. London: Routledge.

Riley JC (1987) *The Eighteenth-century Campaign to Avoid Disease*. London: Macmillan.

Rosen G (1958) *A History of Public Health*. Baltimore, MD: Johns Hopkins University Press.

Shapiro A-L (1985) *Housing the Poor of Paris, 1850–1902*. Madison, WI: University of Wisconsin Press.

Wanless D (2004) *Securing Good Health for the Whole Population*. London: The Stationery Office.

Wohl AS (1983) *Endangered Lives: Public Health in Victorian Britain*. London: Methuen.

Wrigley E and Schofield R (1989) *The Population History of England 1541–1871: A Reconstruction* (2nd edn). Cambridge: Cambridge University Press.

3 Public health in the West since 1800: The responses

Martin Gorsky

Overview

Having seen the challenges to health posed by rapid industrialization and urbanization, the aim now is to understand the responses of local and national governments. These laid the foundations of public health today, not just through laws, institutions and professions, but also through the establishment of the principles that health was a public good and that government had a duty to intervene in maintaining it. First, we present some basic facts about public health policies, drawing on the examples of leading industrialized nations of the nineteenth century – Britain, Germany, France and the United States. Next, we focus on explanations for why the state took these unprecedented actions: after all, it was entering a field previously considered a matter of individual choice. It is tempting to view this history as a 'march of progress', but we will also ask whether this reading is appropriate, or whether there were other directions that might have been taken.

Learning objectives

After working through this chapter you will be able to:

- describe some key policy developments in the field of public health in some Western industrialized nations in the nineteenth century
- review and synthesize historical explanations for these developments
- critically analyse primary and secondary sources related to public health policies

Key terms

Collectivism political action premised on the interdependence of individuals and the need for local or national intervention to advance the public interest.

Laissez-faire French phrase that loosely translates as 'leave alone', and in politics implies non-intervention in economic life.

Liberalism Political belief founded on the importance of individual liberty, usually understood to include constitutional government, democratic participation, free trade, freedom of expression and religion.

> **Sanitary reform** Nineteenth-century public health movement that championed environmental interventions to address sewerage, refuse and fresh water.

Introduction

The first government programmes to tackle the health risks of urban industrial society included smallpox vaccination, environmental management and other preventive strategies for infectious diseases. Also important were the societies and journals founded to promote specialist expertise in this field of medicine. The first section of this chapter briefly details these developments in the advanced economies, as a prelude to the explanations examined later in the chapter.

The entry of the state

Britain

Britain was a forerunner in creating public health institutions of the central state, although in practice these operated mostly through local government. Officials and public health doctors were given powers and sanctions to enforce sanitary reform and preventive measures over citizens' lives. Key events included:

- 1834: Poor Law Amendment Act – appointment of local medical officers to care for paupers.
- 1848: Public Health Act – creation of General Board of Health (until 1854) to enforce establishment of local Boards of Health in towns with high mortality. Boards to have tax-raising powers to cover sanitation, appointment of Medical Officer of Health (MOH), regulation of trades and poor housing, removal of nuisances (i.e. waste, garbage), provision of parks, bathhouses etc.
- 1853: Vaccination Act (smallpox) – compulsory for infants up to 3 months of age.
- 1855: Appointment of first Chief Medical Officer (John Simon).
- 1864, 1866, 1869: Contagious Diseases Acts – compulsory examination of prostitutes to control sexually transmitted diseases.
- 1867, 1871, 1874: Vaccination Acts (smallpox) – non-compliant parents liable to fines and imprisonment.
- 1872: Public Health Act – creation of sanitary authorities with powers to build isolation hospitals; compulsory to appoint MOHs.
- 1875: Public Health Act – codifies all existing sanitary legislation and makes adoption of it compulsory.
- 1875: University of Cambridge institutes first English Diploma in Public Health.
- 1889: Notification Act – sanitary authorities permitted to enforce notification of infectious diseases.

Germany

Germany cannot be considered a nation with central government until political unification in 1871. Before this it was a collection of states, principalities and city-states, of which Prussia was the largest single territory. At first, then, public health action took place at the level of states or cities. However, Germany saw the first full codification of public health law. Prussia moved even earlier than Britain to create public health structures in local government, and consequently Germany is considered to have been authoritarian and centrist in health policy.

- 1779–1825: Publication of Johann Frank's six-volume *System of Complete Medical Police*, a blueprint for public health law to cover individual behaviour 'from womb to tomb'; however, it was never fully adopted.
- 1807 onwards: Compulsory smallpox vaccination introduced in some German cities and states.
- 1817: Prussia appoints *Kreisphysickus*, a local public health doctor in cities and rural districts responsible for forensic medicine and sanitary inspection.
- 1850s–1870s: Local action leads to the development of sanitary infrastructure in Berlin and Munich.
- 1867: Formation of Society of German Hygienists.
- 1873: Formation of central *Reichsgesundheitsamt* [Imperial Hygiene Department] with duties of statistics collection, infectious diseases control, smallpox vaccination and regulation of medical profession.
- 1874: Imperial Vaccination Law – universal, free, compulsory vaccination and revaccination at age 11.
- 1896: Compulsory notification of smallpox.

France

Although France took the intellectual lead in public health theory during the early nineteenth century, it lagged behind Britain and Germany in setting up strong central institutions and compulsory preventive measures. This was probably because French politics was infused with a stronger commitment to liberal individualism and respect for private property. The experience of Revolution in 1789, with its sequels of violent Terror and despotic rule by Napoleon Bonaparte, had made the state wary of heavy-handed interventions that might prompt resistance. Again, then, action mostly took place at the local level.

- 1794: Institution of Chair of Hygiene, University of Paris, leads to development of *parti d'hygiene* (doctors and researchers interested in public health).
- 1802: Founding of *Conseil de Salubrité de la Seine* (Board of Health for Paris) to advise on pollution and sanitation, but with no powers of enforcement.
- 1822 onwards: more *Conseils de Salubrité* founded, including Lyon (1822), Marseille (1825) and Bordeaux (1831), although lack of powers makes them largely ineffective.
- 1829: Foundation of journal *Annales d'Hygiène Publique et Medicine Légale*.
- 1848: Public Health Law – a health council to be appointed in each department, canton and *arrondissement*, although few worked effectively.
- 1870s: Bureau of Health and Hygiene created within Ministry of the Interior.

- 1893: Medical Assistance Act – obliges departments and communes to provide medical assistance to the destitute.
- 1902: Public Hygiene Act – empowers communes to arrange municipal water supply for each inhabited dwelling, paid for by local taxes. Smallpox vaccination made compulsory; notification of infectious diseases.

United States of America

In the USA, politicians cherished notions of individual liberty even more highly than in France and harboured great suspicion of empowering federal (i.e. national) institutions. Public health action therefore mostly took place at the level of the state and city where the effects of mass migration and rapid urbanization were being felt.

- 1798–1805: Early urban Boards of Health appointed, including Boston (1798), New Orleans (1804) and New York City (1805) but with limited powers and typically only active during epidemics.
- 1855: Formation of first State Board of Health in Louisiana.
- 1866: New York Metropolitan Board of Health with powers of enforcement covering sanitary inspection, drainage, food safety, inspection of offensive trades, collection of statistics; provides model for other cities and states.
- 1869 onwards: Formation of State Boards of Health, including Massachusetts (1869), California (1870) and Illinois (1877).
- 1872: Formation of American Public Health Association.
- 1879–1883: Temporary National Board of Health, during yellow fever epidemic.
- 1902: Formation of federal Public Health and Marine Hospital Service (renamed US Public Health Service in 1915) as advisory body to manage immigration.

Explaining change

Britain, Germany, France and the United States therefore took different routes to public health reform, moving quickly or slowly to central organization, and striking their own balance between compulsion and liberty. In this brief overview, we do not have time to explore all the reasons for these differences, which are extremely complex. Instead, the discussion that follows will try to find some general explanations, not for the differences, but for the similarities between the nations that piloted public health reform.

Economic history: A case of market failure?

At the broadest level, we may explain the entry of the state into public health as a response to the problems thrown up by the Industrial Revolution. The economist Karl Polanyi argued that these problems were caused by excessive faith in the power of the free markets that characterized the first industrial era. Here is how he describes the situation in the early nineteenth century:

> The effects on the lives of the people were awful beyond description ... the labouring people had been crowded together in new places of desolation, the so-called

> industrial towns ... the country folk had been dehumanized into slum dwellers ...
> large parts of the country were rapidly disappearing under the slack and scrap heaps
> vomited forth from the 'satanic mills' ... Indeed human society would have been
> annihilated but for protective counter-moves which blunted the action of the self-
> destructive mechanism.
>
> (Polanyi, 1944/2001, pp. 41–2, 79)

Public health, then, was one of these 'counter-moves'. Polanyi thought that because
such initiatives had taken place in several different countries at roughly the same time
they could not be attributed to any political party or belief. Instead, they were a prag-
matic response to problems that legislators of all different political stripes could see.

Thus, this argument gives us a very general explanation: states stepped in when markets failed. However, it cannot explain the timing of legislation and the form this took.

Intellectual history: Science and infectious disease

The next step in understanding public health reform is therefore to consider the science that shaped the new practices. As we saw in Chapter 2, the major breakthrough
of modern medicine – Pasteur's germ theory of disease – did not gain acceptance until
the final third of the nineteenth century. However, there were several other key scientific developments that underpinned public health interventions.

Jenner and vaccination

In the 1790s, Edward Jenner, an English country doctor, revolutionized the treatment
for smallpox. Smallpox was an aerial-borne viral disease, whose acute form, *Variola
major*, had a fatality rate of up to 30 per cent. Symptoms included fever, muscular pains
and headache, followed by a body rash ('pox') that developed into pustules, leaving
survivors badly scarred. It had long been a practice of Asian traditional medicine to
inoculate against smallpox by scratching a small amount of vesicular fluid under the
skin. In the eighteenth century, Western doctors had adopted this therapy, using a lancet (a small surgical blade) to cut the arm. This proved dangerous because of risks of
infection through miscalculation of the dose.

Jenner was a London-educated doctor trained in the new practices of clinical observation. Back in Gloucestershire he noticed that local dairymaids regularly contracted a
mild disease called 'cowpox' from milking cows, and that this conferred immunity from
smallpox. He therefore conducted experiments to determine whether inoculation
with the weaker cowpox pus would be effective against smallpox. The hypothesis was
proven: Jenner had discovered a safer inoculation technique, quickly renamed 'vaccination' (after *vacca*, Latin for cow). The way was now open for the mass programmes that
would eventually lead to global eradication of smallpox in 1977.

Miasma and the theory of contagion

A great irony of public health history is that the early campaigns for improved drainage,
sewerage and clean water were built on faulty science. The belief that dirt, garbage
and excrement were a breeding ground for disease predated germ theory, and drew
instead on the concept of 'miasma', first articulated in Ancient Greece. The idea was

that putrefying matter emitted poisons (miasms) into the air that were carriers of disease. Scientists were divided on exactly how this led to infection. One explanation was 'zymosis', a process by which aerial-borne poisons proliferated in the bloodstream rather like the fermentation of yeast cells. These then became the causal agents of the 'zymotic diseases' (see Figure 2.4). Miasmatic theory was strengthened by empirical observation of the proximity of infections to unhygienic spaces. (Remember the 'filthy courts and close places' of the Bilston cholera epidemic in Chapter 1.) Thus a programme of sanitary reform was launched before a coherent understanding of bacterial transmission was available.

Epidemiology and environment: Theory

The foundations of epidemiology were being laid in this period through the collection of vital statistics and census data. Developments took place early in France, where statistical techniques, dubbed the *méthode numérique*, were applied to health. These represent a first attempt systematically to test long-standing theories about the relationship between place and disease.

Exercise 3.1: Villermé and differential mortality in Paris

The analysis in the source below is treasured by historians of epidemiology because it represents a milestone in understanding. Louis-René Villermé was a leading practitioner of the *méthode numérique*, and in 1824 he was exploring statistical associations between mortality and environmental factors in the different *arrondissements* (districts) of Paris. Drawing on then current theories of links between environment and health he introduced variables such as building types, wind direction, elevation and sunlight. None of these yielded significant correlation. He also tried two other variables.

Table 3.1 Mortality and social conditions in Paris, 1817–1821

Arrondissement	Mortality rate (per 1000)	Overcrowding (%)	Poverty (%)
2nd	16	75	7
3rd	17	55	11
1st	17	57	11
4th	17	59	15
6th	19	62	21
5th	19	46	22
7th	19	82	22
11th	20	55	19
10th	20	53	23
9th	23	60	31
8th	23	46	32
12th	23	64	38

Note: mortality = deaths per 1000 (author's calculations); overcrowding = percentage of surface area occupied by buildings; poverty = percentage of poor families with untaxed property.

Source: Data from La Berge (1992, pp. 59–64).

1 What question was Villermé asking?
2 What did his results show?

Feedback

Villermé wanted to establish whether social conditions affected mortality rates using a simple visual comparison.

The degree of 'overcrowding' displayed no obvious relationship with death rates, but there was an almost exact correlation between levels of wealth and mortality. Villermé had demonstrated for the first time a social gradient in mortality according to affluence.

In England, the establishment of the Registrar General's Office led to the appointment in 1838 of William Farr as 'compiler of abstracts' (the first official medical statistician). Farr developed the analysis of cause of death statistics, used census data to refine indicators for overcrowding and like Villermé observed differential mortality. He explained this from a miasmatist standpoint, assuming the disadvantage of the urban poor was due to insanitary living conditions.

Epidemiology and environment: Field investigations

At the same time, the recurrence of epidemic cholera had prompted two English doctors, William Budd in Bristol and John Snow in London, to conduct the fieldwork that finally proved it was a waterborne infectious disease, transmitted by the faecal–oral route. Budd had initially worked on typhoid (salmonella poisoning) and had deduced from observation of a small epidemic that polluted water was the cause. As Bristol's Medical Officer of Health from 1849 he initiated sanitary reform to prevent typhoid and also cholera, which he believed to have the same aetiology. This significantly reduced local mortality in the 1866 cholera outbreak.

John Snow is better known because he promoted his theories more successfully to the London intelligentsia. Snow had originally speculated about faecal–oral transmission direct to the alimentary canal following his first-hand observations of the 1831 epidemic. After cholera's return in 1848–1849, he built his case by comparative analysis of mortality rates in areas supplied by different water companies and river sources. The 1853–1854 outbreak offered a chance to confirm the hypothesis, and Snow conducted a systematic study of water quality and cholera deaths in Soho, central London. He famously persuaded the local vestry (parish council) to remove the pump handle from the fresh water well in Broad Street, which he believed to be the source of infection. Mortality fell and this theatrical gesture vindicated Snow's ideas (although the disease had already peaked by then!). A local vicar, Henry Whitehead, then confirmed the theory by tracing the first case to a cesspool, which inspection showed was seeping through decayed brickwork into the Broad Street well. Even then, many refused to abandon the conventional wisdom about miasma. In 1866, however, William Farr discovered that differential mortality in London correlated to water company supplies, which persuaded him to abandon miasma theory and support Snow's argument. The case for sanitary reform had now been convincingly made.

The bacteriological 'revolution'

By the late nineteenth century, the laboratory began to loom larger in the scientific understanding of diseases, following Pasteur's work. Now the quest was on to identify the role of microorganisms in disease aetiology, using microscopy and new techniques of cultivation. Pasteur himself demonstrated the therapeutic potential of immunization using less virulent strains of the pathogenic microbes, when his rabies vaccine was successfully trialled in 1885. Meanwhile, researchers identified the causal role of different microbes, most famously Robert Koch's work on anthrax (1876), tuberculosis (1882) and cholera (1883), and Laveran's on malaria (1880). Others found the organisms responsible for typhoid, diphtheria, tetanus, plague and dysentery. However, before 1900 these discoveries were rarely translated into usable therapies, with Koch's unsuccessful launch of 'tuberculin' as a cure for tuberculosis the greatest disappointment. Only in the mid-1890s did two developments of real significance for public health occur, with the first uses of a diphtheria serum antitoxin and of a typhoid vaccine.

In considering these breakthroughs, we must not assume that new discoveries, however brilliant, were automatically recognized and adopted. Historians of medicine stress that the impact of any scientific innovation is contingent on other factors, quite apart from the natural reluctance of scientists to abandon theories on which they have staked their careers. Even with the germ theory, research by Michael Worboys (2000) into the medical debates surrounding the action of microbes and their implications for preventive medicine shows that there was no instant 'revolutionary' switch to a new consensus. Therefore, we also need to consider the political, economic and social context in which ideas were launched and which determined how quickly they were picked up.

Political history: Setting the reform agenda

As a first step, we need to turn from long-term developments in the history of ideas to the short-term history of events. How, in practice, was the reform agenda set?

Individuals and social investigation

A number of key individuals had great influence on public opinion and on policy-makers. They achieved this through publication of detailed reports, mostly commissioned by national or municipal governments, which documented the relationship between urban conditions and health. Of these the work of the British lawyer and civil servant Edwin Chadwick, *Report on the Sanitary Condition of the Labouring Population of Great Britain* (1842), is probably the best known, because it prompted national public health legislation. Other examples are Villermé's *Survey of the Physical and Moral Conditions of the Workers Employed in the Cotton, Wool and Silk Factories* (1840), which precipitated French child labour legislation, and in the USA, John Griscom's *The Sanitary Condition of the Labouring Population in New York* (1845), and Lemuel Shattuck's *Report of the Sanitary Commission of Massachusetts* (1850). In addition to empirical data on urban public health these texts reflected the contemporary mindset, which saw hygiene as moral and religious improvement, or appealed to evangelical or humanitarian impulses.

Rather different was a German study of 1848 by the pathologist Rudolf Virchow, *Communications about the Typhus Epidemic in Upper Silesia*, which explicitly linked disease to poverty, and by extension to lack of political rights. Virchow concluded: 'the future is therefore very easy and simple: education, liberty and prosperity ... free and unlimited democracy'. This was the first great statement that a public health doctor must also be an 'attorney for the poor', and that the job was unavoidably political. Virchow wrote: 'Medicine is a social science, and politics is nothing more than medicine on a large scale.' (Virchow, 1848).

Exercise 3.2: Edwin Chadwick's *Report on the Sanitary Condition of the Labouring Population of Great Britain*

Study the following extract, which comes from Chadwick's concluding chapter, and then answer the questions that follow. His report was based on an extensive survey of the health and living conditions of the poor, compiled through questionnaires and requests submitted to about 2000 people. Its text consisted largely of the resulting first-hand descriptions by local doctors, poor law officials, schoolteachers and others. It then suggested what might be done to improve the situation.

'After as careful an examination of the evidence collected as I have been enabled to make, I beg leave to recapitulate the chief conclusions ...

First ... that the various forms of epidemic, endemic and other disease caused, or aggravated, or propagated chiefly amongst the labouring classes by atmospheric impurities produced by decomposing animal and vegetable substances, by damp and filth, and close and overcrowded dwellings prevail amongst the population ...

That such disease, wherever its attacks are frequent, is always found in connexion with the physical circumstances above specified, and that where these circumstances are removed by drainage, proper cleansing, better ventilation and other means of diminishing atmospheric impurity, the frequency and intensity of such disease is abated ...

That high prosperity in respect of employment and wages, and various and abundant food, have afforded to the labouring classes no exemptions from attacks of epidemic disease, which have been as frequent and as fatal in periods of commercial and manufacturing prosperity as in any others.

That the annual loss of life from filth and bad ventilation are greater than the loss from death or wounds in any wars in which the country has been engaged in modern times.

That of the 43,000 cases of widowhood, and 112,000 cases of destitute orphanage relieved from the poor's rates in England and Wales alone, it appears that the greatest proportion of deaths of heads of families occurred from the above specified and other removable causes; that their ages were under 45 years; that is to say, 13 years below the natural probabilities of life as shown by the experience of the whole population of Sweden.

That, measuring the loss of working ability amongst large classes by the instances of gain, even from the incomplete arrangements for the removal of noxious influences from places of work or from abodes, that this loss cannot be less than eight or ten years.

That the younger population, bred up under noxious physical agencies, is inferior in physical organisation and in general health to a population preserved from the presence of such agencies.

That the population so exposed is less susceptible of moral influences, and the effects of education are more transient than with a healthy population.

That these adverse circumstances tend to produce an adult population short-lived, improvident, reckless, and intemperate, and with habitual avidity for sensual gratifications.

That defective town cleansing fosters habits of the most abject degradation and tends to the demoralisation of large numbers of human beings, who subsist by means of what they find amidst the noxious filth accumulated in neglected streets and bye-places.

That the expenses of local public works are in general unequally and unfairly assessed, oppressively and uneconomically collected, by separate collections, wastefully expended in separate and inefficient operations by unskilled and practically irresponsible officers ...

And that the removal of noxious physical circumstances, and the promotion of civic, household, and personal cleanliness are necessary to the improvement of the moral condition of the population; for that sound morality and refinement in manners and health are not long found co-existent with filthy habits amongst any class of the community.'

(Chadwick, 1842, pp. 422–5)

1 How did Chadwick explain the public health problems he had described?
2 How did he make the case for sanitary reform?
3 How convincing do you find his arguments?

Feedback

1 Chadwick explains morbidity and mortality using the theory of miasma, which assumes that aerial emanations from putrefying refuse are the cause of disease and that removal through sanitary measures will diminish risk. He claims that wealth and nutritional status cannot be relevant causal agents because epidemics can strike during phases of buoyant economic growth.

2 His case for reform is not based on humanitarianism. Instead, he emphasizes the benefit to the economy from increasing years of productive labour. He also places great emphasis on moral issues, arguing that poor environmental conditions can shape behaviour, by encouraging people to 'live for the moment' and indulge in sensory pleasures. Thus sanitary reform will foster personal and civic decency. Finally, he stresses that leaving these matters to the smallest and most local units of government is inefficient and inequitable in terms of cost distribution.

3 With the benefit of subsequent knowledge about the relationship between economic growth and mortality decline, we may find Chadwick's dismissal of wealth and nutritional status unconvincing. From an ethical or human rights standpoint, we may find it surprising that he rests his case so heavily on economic grounds. We may also read his discussion of 'moralising' the poor as a reflection of his Victorian middle-class prejudices. However, it is worth considering that as a rhetorical strategy, these arguments probably carried weight with the people Chadwick had to convince to spend money. And while we may find his attitudes alien to our own, we should perhaps consider whether there are elements of paternalism and moralizing in contemporary health promotion efforts, for example relating to alcohol, drugs or smoking?

The shock effect of 'King Cholera'

Another factor that set the agenda in the short term was epidemic cholera. In most cases, the causation was not direct, and indeed the nineteenth-century death toll from cholera was not as high as that of other diseases, such as pulmonary tuberculosis. However, because the early epidemics saw such concentrated mortality and high case fatality, cholera had a real 'shock effect'. Here is how the historian Asa Briggs put it:

'Whenever it threatened European countries ... it tested the efficiency and resilience of local administrative structure. It exposed relentlessly political, social and moral shortcomings.' Cholera was 'a catalyst of public opinion, an ally in the service of the "sanitary reformers"' (Briggs, 1961, pp. 79, 86).

Exercise 3.3: Visualizing the impact of cholera

To gain a sense of this shock effect, study the cartoon below, which appeared in an American periodical in 1883, during one of the late nineteenth-century pandemics.

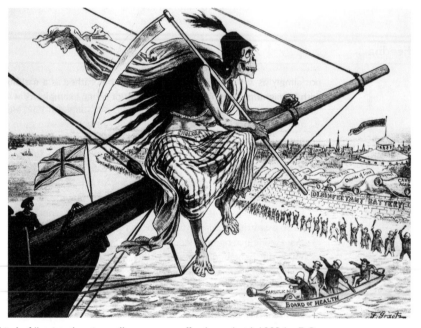

Figure 3.1 'The kind of "assisted emigrant" we cannot afford to admit', 1883 by F. Graetz

Source: Puck, July 18, 1883

You may find it helpful to know that the setting is the Battery area, at the southern tip of Manhattan Island, New York. The building with the flag is Castle Clinton, which from 1855 to 1890 was America's immigrant processing centre, and the 1880s was a period in which migration to America was escalating. Note that an assisted emigrant was one whose government paid their fare to help them leave the country.

• With these points in mind, what does the cartoon tell us about attitudes towards cholera and to public health?

Feedback

We need to be careful not to assume a single image can represent widely held atti-tudes. Nonetheless, there is a good chance that in choosing the motifs and narrative for the cartoon, the artist hoped to express ideas that resonated with the public. Bearing in mind that everyone will 'read' this slightly differently, here is one possible interpreta-tion: The emotional power comes from the frightening depiction of cholera as the 'grim reaper', whose huge scythe will decimate his victims. The sailors on the British ship are unaware of his presence, and his bare feet are poised on the rope like an acrobat's. The message is that the cholera is a supple and elusive threat. Public health is portrayed through a military metaphor, as a powerful defence against this menace. Bottles of disinfectant point like cannons at the ship, and the officials of New York's Board of Health can see the danger, unlike the heedless sailors. The remedy is carbolic acid (today known as phenol), a derivative of coal tar, whose antiseptic properties led to its use in surgery and as a general disinfectant. Public health officials and the science that supported them are therefore viewed positively, as America's first line of protection.

Finally, note how the disease is depicted as something 'foreign', an embodied 'other', whose clothing and headgear denote Middle Eastern origins. Cholera is represented not simply as a global hazard for humanity, but rather as a national threat associated with immigrants. You may be able to think of other examples of when an epidemic has led to the demonizing of a minority group. For example, in the 1980s gay men suffered similar opprobrium in the early phase of the HIV/AIDS pandemic, while the 2002–2003 SARS outbreak in North America saw the blaming of Chinese communities.

Political history: Changing nature of the state

So far, we have examined the need for reform, the science that underpinned it, and some of the factors that put public health on the political agenda. To complete our understanding of how all this translated into policy, we now consider the nature and functions of the state, whether at local or national levels, and changing ideas about its role as the era of popular democracy and modern party politics dawned.

Capacity: The growth in size and function

Information and argument alone could not have affected change if the state had not had the capacity to implement new policies. The nineteenth century saw the growth in size and activity of the government in several areas, not just health. State schooling systems were emerging, with, for example, Prussia implementing compulsory attendance in 1819, and each commune in France obliged from 1833 to open a public elementary school. County police forces were set up in Britain in 1839, while early American police departments included Boston (1838) and New York (1845). In Britain, the numbers of people employed by the state increased from 250,000 in 1850 to almost a million by 1900, and this reflected a simultaneous growth in wealth and tax receipts: public spend-ing in 1900 was 14 per cent of gross national product (Pugh, 1994, pp. 56–9). So, the emergence of modern public health was part of a bigger growth in state activity.

Indeed, in his theory of the 'Revolution in Victorian Government', Oliver MacDonagh (1958) argued that social reforms addressing issues such as factory conditions, educa-tion and health had a built-in dynamic of expansion. First, problems were identified and state involvement started on a small scale, perhaps with grants to civil society organizations or laws to regulate the private sector, with related inspection systems. Then, bureaucratic expertise and control grew slowly, laws were refined and strengthened, spending increased, and gradually the state came to take the lead.

Democracy: The emergence of mass electorates and party politics

The idea of a political right to health for those who could not afford it had first been articulated in 1790–1791, during the French Revolution. This was when rule by king and aristocracy had been swept away, to be replaced by constitutional government exercised by elected representatives. The century that followed saw major change in the nature of the state, with the extension of the 'suffrage' – the right to vote. Admittedly, this was a slow process, and women did not generally gain this right until the early twentieth century. But in Britain, for example, middle-class men had gained the vote in 1832, the urban working class in 1867 and agricultural labourers in 1884–1885.

So can we say that the right to vote led on to the right to health, and thus to public health reforms? As we will see in Chapter 10 this would be an oversimplification, because the people have not always wanted the health reforms that their leaders proposed! However, it is striking that in Britain, soon after the Reform Act of 1867, a Public Health Act (1872) was passed. This was also the moment when health entered the programmes of political parties, as part of their electoral appeal. For example, in a speech in Manchester in 1872, the British Conservative Party leader, Benjamin Disraeli, declared 'sanitas sanitatum, omnia sanitas' [health, of health, all is health], and argued that 'the first consideration of a Minister should be the health of the people' (cited in Kebbel, 1882, pp. 511–12).

Ideology: The changing nature of liberalism

The championing of public health was not just a matter of pragmatism on the part of vote-hungry politicians. It also marked a changing acceptance by politicians and lawmakers of the proper role of the state in people's lives. In 1905, the writer A.V. Dicey described this as a transition from 'laissez-faire' (leaving alone) to 'collectivism' (intervention by national or local government in the interests of the public). He thought this was most extreme in England because of its democratic electorate and strong central state. The British Liberal Party politician, Joseph Chamberlain (1836–1914), put it like this:

> Now Government is the organised expression of the wishes and wants of the people, and under these circumstances let us cease to regard it with suspicion. Suspicion is the product of an older time – of circumstances which have long since disappeared. Now it is our business to extend its functions, and to see in what ways its operations can be usefully enlarged.
>
> (quoted in Boyd, 1914, p. 164)

Social history: Class, knowledge and power

Until now, the story this chapter has told is one of progress. In brief, it goes like this: economic development led to serious social problems, which were gradually set right by a combination of better science, astute campaigning and democratic politics. But is there a danger that we are telling a 'Whig' history of public health, a history that assumes Western liberal societies were marching inexorably forward to the betterment of their populations?

A more sceptical view was proposed by the philosopher-historian Michel Foucault, who claimed that public health interventions should be understood as an aspect of 'biopolitics' – that is, modern society's increasing control over the body 'as a factor of productive force, of labor power' (Foucault, 1974/1994, p. 137). His argument was that capitalist production, urbanization and the social unrest sparked by the French Revolution created a new situation in which the bodies of the poor became politically important. Foucault contended that public health primarily benefited the privileged, protecting them from the threat of epidemic disease and ensuring that the workforce stayed healthy. This was hardly collectivism.

Let us finish with another dissenting verdict, from Christopher Hamlin, who in 1998 caused a stir by writing a revisionist history of Edwin Chadwick and public health reform in Britain. Delving into the publications of contemporary writers who addressed the same social issues as Chadwick, he concluded that environmental reform had not been the only choice for public health policy.

Exercise 3.4: The greatest 'technical fix' in history?

Read the following extract from the introduction to Hamlin's book where he sets out his argument, and then answer the questions that follow.

'Consider the kind of public health that arose in Britain, one preoccupied with water and wastes. It is difficult to acknowledge a need to explain this, for it remains a central and uncontroversial part of public health. The water and sewage technologies the sanitarians developed quickly became one of the most widely diffused technological complexes in human history. They so exemplify development and decency (not to mention health) that many of us judge places mainly on "sanitary" grounds: be the inhabitants dull, rude, even brutal, so long as they have restrooms they are civilized.

If public health is understood in this way, its history is pretty well done. Here Chadwick the discoverer is but the vehicle for truth. Carried on the current of empirical social science, he can do no other in leading the way to sanitary salvation. Our only job will be to chart that salvation in town after town.

The vision of the inexorable progress of science and health is usually founded in an appeal to "conditions", the idea that public health activity is driven by public health need. Filling our narratives are overflowing privies and windowless cellars ... Accompanying them are death tolls of epidemic diseases ascribed to these conditions. Often historians move from descriptions of such conditions to the conclusion that those conditions demanded remedies and that they were therefore provided, more or less expeditiously. Yet the historian's imperative has no teeth. Of course conditions were deplorable, but their deplorability tells us nothing about who responded to them and how. The need was not always met; the responsibility had to be recognized and acted upon. Not everybody, not in Britain, not in Europe, not in the rest of the world, not then, not now, had or has drains and water ... The recognition that conditions do not determine responses is necessary if we are to avoid falling under the rhetorical spell cast by sanitarians a century and a half ago.

...the early Victorians invented one public health among many. Their sanitary movement was not a systematic campaign to eliminate excess mortality. Its concern was with *some aspects* of the health of *some* people: working-class men of working age. Women, infants, children, and the aged were largely ignored ... It tended, moreover, to represent those men in terms of their houses, streets, drains, or towns. The condition of Chadwick's man could be reduced to the rate at which his sewage flowed down a tube and the volume of air that passed his nose, and secondly to the tidiness of his cottage ... but only slightly to the temperature of his dwelling, and the adequacy of his clothing, and the quality and quantity of the aliment that vanished down his esphagus.

Yet there was another position, a position which viewed as pathological the totality of social and economic conditions in which the Industrial Revolution had left many poor people. This is not simply a position in principle. It was occupied, but by poorly organized groups who often disagreed with one another on fundamental issues ... To members of these groups, the idea that some facet of industrialization and urbanization – whether overwork, trade cycles, or tariffs – killed people was by no means a comfortable belief; it was on the contrary absolutely unacceptable. There was here the raw material for making health as prominent a criterion for the assessment of public policy as, say, economics has become. That did not happen. Chadwick and company rejected work, wages and food to focus on water and filth, arguably the greatest "technical fix" in history.'

Source: Hamlin (1998, pp. 7–10, 12–13)

1 What criticisms does Hamlin make of previous public health histories?
2 How convincing is his argument that there might have been an alternative approach to public health?

Feedback

1 Hamlin argues we are so accustomed to modern standards of sanitary hygiene that we do not think critically enough about how they came about. We simply assume that they were an automatic response to the problems of the time, which Chadwick was the first to diagnose. But a fuller consideration of debates about public health in this period tells us that both the diagnosis and remedy were hotly contested. Looked at in this way we can see that the 'sewers and drains' approach was partial and selective. Its main concern was with the economic productivity of adult working-class men, and it ignored other vital issues, such as occupational diseases and poor nutrition. Better sanitation led to some improvements, but it did not fundamentally challenge the inequalities that determined much ill health.

2 In response to Hamlin we might reasonably argue that amidst the raging free-market capitalism of the industrial West, there was never a realistic possibility that such redistributive policies could have occurred. At least Chadwick deserves credit for what he did achieve. But maybe that misses Hamlin's main point, which is to make us aware that health policies are often the outcome of power struggles in which notions of human rights and social justice take the back seat.

Summary

The subject of this chapter has been the growth of government intervention in public health exemplified by four leading industrial nations of the nineteenth century, viewed widely as the forerunners of reform. The reforms they implemented are remembered chiefly as environmental interventions: major programmes of urban infrastructural renewal that significantly affected mortality from enteric diseases. Other elements of reform included: fostering the academic specialty of public health and providing it with an administrative location; promoting smallpox vaccination; and the isolation and notification of infectious diseases. In explaining this it is necessary, but not sufficient, to note the contexts of urban squalor that accompanied industrialization and the developing science of infectious diseases. Also important were the changing nature of liberal democratic states, and the individuals whose investigations and advocacy set the agenda for change. We have also seen that the making of modern public health was not driven by concerns for equity and rights. Ideas about economic efficiency and moral reform also mattered in determining the nature of change. In the next chapter, we consider the role played by the developing health professions in the ongoing evolution of public health.

References and further reading

Baldwin P (1999) *Contagion and the State in Europe, 1830–1930*. New York: Cambridge University Press.

Boyd C (ed) (1914) *Mr Chamberlain's Speeches*, Vol. I. London: Constable.

Briggs A (1961) Cholera and society in the nineteenth century, *Past and Present*, 19 (1): 76–96.

Chadwick E (1842/1965) *Report on the Sanitary Condition of the Labouring Population of Great Britain* (edited by MW Flinn). Edinburgh: Edinburgh University Press.

Dicey A (1905/1963) *Lectures on the Relation Between Law & Public Opinion in England During the Nineteenth Century* (2nd edn). London: Macmillan.

Duffy J (1990) *The Sanitarians: A History of American Public Health*. Urbana, IL: University of Illinois Press.

Foucault M (1974/1994) The birth of social medicine, in *Power: Essential Works of Foucault, 1954–1984* (edited by J Faubion), pp. 134–56. London: Penguin.

Goubert J-P (1989) *The Conquest of Water: The Advent of Health in the Industrial Age*. Princeton, NJ: Princeton University Press.

Hamlin C (1998) *Public Health and Social Justice in the Age of Chadwick, Britain, 1800–1854*. Cambridge: Cambridge University Press.

Kebbel T (ed) (1882) *Selected Speeches of the Late Right Honourable the Earl of Beaconsfield*, Vol II. London: Longmans, Green and co.

La Berge A (1992) *Mission and Method: The Early Nineteenth Century French Public Health Movement*. Cambridge: Cambridge University Press.

Macdonagh O (1958) The nineteenth century revolution in government: A reappraisal, *Historical Journal*, I: 52–67.

Polanyi K (1944/2001) *The Great Transformation: The Political and Economic Origins of Our Time* (2nd edn). Boston, MA: Beacon Press.

Porter D (1999) *Health, Civilization and the State*. London: Routledge.

Pugh M (1994) *State and Society: British Political and Social History 1870–1922*. London: Edward Arnold.

Russell G (1911) *One Look Back*. London: Wells Gardner, Darton and Co.

Virchow R (1848) 'Der Armenarzt' (The Charity Doctor), *Die Medizinische Reform*, and (1848) *Mittheilungen uber die Oberschlesien herrschende Typhus-Epidemie*, Berlin: Reimer, in Rather L (1990) *A Commentary on the Medical Writings of Rudolf Virchow, 1843–1901*. San Francisco, CA: Norman.

Worboys M (2000) *Spreading Germs: Disease Theories and Medical Practice in Britain, 1865–1900*. Cambridge: Cambridge University Press.

4 The development of the health professions

Virginia Berridge

Overview

This chapter moves from the focus on public health conditions and responses to look at the role of the health professions. Public health developed as a professional activity, as an occupation, alongside more general professionalization in health and medicine. The nineteenth century saw the formation of distinct boundaries between regular and irregular medical practitioners, between orthodox medicine, 'quacks' and commercial practitioners. Formal professional structures replaced the chaotic regulation of earlier times. Distinct boundaries between primary care physicians and specialists emerged in Britain but not in all countries. Public health also established itself as a medical profession, but public health doctors did not have the same status as other doctors. Access to regular health care remained limited and other health workers such as druggists and pharmacists played an important role in providing it. A gendered division of labour in health care emerged, which, by the early years of the twentieth century, was formalized in new nursing and midwifery professions.

Learning objectives

After working through this chapter, you will be able to:

- describe how the professionalization of health occupations developed during the nineteenth and early twentieth centuries
- use primary sources to identify and explain the factors involved in shaping the role of different professions and the position of public health practitioners
- distinguish between the role of the different health professions and the gendered division of health care labour

Key terms

Apothecary Originally a seller of remedies, but later in the UK became an organized occupation that joined with the surgeons in the early nineteenth century as a prototype general practitioner.

Druggist A dispenser of drugs. This was the term in common use before the more professionalized term of 'pharmacist' came into use in the nineteenth century.

Gender Term referring to the socially constructed roles, behaviours, activities and attributes that a given society considers appropriate for men and women.

General practitioner Primary health care practitioner who in the UK came to act as 'gatekeeper' filtering access to specialist hospital care.

Global South Refers to nations that have not diversified or are currently in the process of diversifying economically and industrially in a manner that would support the development of the state, access to resources and welfare structures common in Western Europe or North America. The global South includes much of Asia and Latin America, most of Africa, and is related to the terms 'developing world' and 'Third World'.

Midwife Health care worker who provides care to women during pregnancy, labour and birth. Midwives became subordinate to medically qualified practitioners by the early twentieth century although originally more autonomous.

Nurse Health care worker usually subordinate to the doctor and, in hospital, to the medical consultant. Often performed menial tasks in relation to health care, associated with 'women's work'.

Patent medicine Term used to describe commercial medicine or proprietary medicines, sold over the counter in standardized form. Many of these medicines were not actually covered by patents.

Pharmacist Professional responsible for the dispensing and selling of drugs to customers. Pharmacy was on the boundary between commercial medicine and shopkeeping and a professional activity.

Primary health care Health care provided by general practitioners or by health care personnel based in the local community. Primary health care came on the agenda in both developed and developing countries, in the latter in particular after the Alma Ata declaration in 1978. It was connected with the rising costs of specialist hospital-based care but also the view that health care closer to the individual and community would be more effective.

Social medicine A new discipline that aimed to integrate a wide variety of disciplines and variables into the study of ill-health and into social action. In part inspired by the impact of social hygiene in Soviet Russia. It aimed to integrate medicine and the social sciences into the study of individuals as social beings and to provide health services that took account of the social dimensions of health.

Introduction

Health can be dealt with at an individual or at a population level. Public health has traditionally operated at the population level; and health care and services provide for individual patients. In this book, we look at how responses have developed in both areas: public health and health services. In this chapter, we examine how different professional groupings established their competence both for individual patient care and for public health. Historically, one of the tensions within public health has been the relationship between its practitioners and primary health care personnel, epitomized by the general practitioner in the UK. The role of gender has also been important for health care and this is shown in the history of nursing and midwifery, where professional occupations, subordinate to medicine, replaced unqualified, yet often skilled, practitioners. This chapter focuses on the UK story; there are cross-national differences. Pharmacists play a bigger role as front-line practitioners in some countries of the global South and there are now policy moves in some Western countries to emphasize their renewed contribution. Public health has been a medical occupation in the UK, although this is not the case in all countries. There have been recent successful moves in the UK to establish what is called multidisciplinary public health. The development of the health professions in the UK is an important example of the historical roots of the tensions between and within the health professions in many countries both in the past and in the present.

Medical practitioners: Divisions in medicine

In Europe and North America, the demand for health care had been met before the nineteenth century by a wide range of healers. Historians have drawn attention to what they call a 'medical marketplace' in which different types of practitioners set out their wares and the patient decided which he or she wanted to purchase. Medicine was patient dominated rather than doctor dominated as it became in the course of the nineteenth century. The orthodox medical profession has often been characterized as marked by a tripartite division into physicians, surgeons and apothecaries, in descending order of status. But in England the occupational structure of medicine was looser and more competitive than in the rest of Europe and divisions between types of practitioner were by no means clear-cut. This division was an ideal transferred from the city-states of Europe. Medical organization in Scotland more closely resembled the European model and there were close links there with the French and Dutch medical professions.

General practice and regulation

Up to the nineteenth century, barbers and barber surgeons offered the greatest range of personal services from beard dying and tooth scraping to blood letting. The barber surgeon was the nearest equivalent in the pre-nineteenth century period to a general practitioner and provided most formal care in towns in Europe. But some apothecaries also began to call themselves 'doctor' by the seventeenth century and the surgeon apothecary is usually seen as the ancestor of the general practitioner. Rank-and-file medical practitioners managed to redefine themselves and the term 'general practitioner' began to be used by about 1820.

The first British national census to include detailed occupational information (1841) showed that regular practitioners – defined in terms of formal qualifications – were outnumbered by irregulars by a ratio of one to three. These irregulars included druggists, who are discussed in relation to pharmacy below. Hospitals offered an arena for self-definition. A hospital position was honorary and unpaid but offered rewards in terms of social contacts and large fees from pupils.

In London, entry to the upper levels of practice was guarded by the Royal Colleges, of Physicians and of Surgeons. These colleges withheld recognition of courses offered by private or provincial medical schools. But change began to occur in the early nineteenth century as pressure mounted from practitioners who were university trained in the Netherlands, Scotland, Ireland and also at University College in London after 1828.

Exercise 4.1

Selected entries from the Provincial Medical Directory of 1847 are provided below. These directories were commercial ventures that preceded the later professional medical register. Read through these entries and answer the questions that follow.

BARRETT, John, Orange-grove, Bath-Surg.; F.R.C.S. (by exam); Surg. To Western Dispensary; to St Michael's Lying-in Charity; to Great Western Railway (Bath District); Vaccinator and Registrar of Births and Deaths for Abbey District.

BATTEN, THOS., Coleford, Monmouthsh.-General Pract; M.R.C.S. 1827; LSA, 1826; Surgeon to eight collieries in the district.

BEASLEY, John, Oadby Blaby, Leicester-Gen.Pract; In practice prior to the Act of 1815.

BEDINGFIELD, James, Stowmarket, Suffolk-Gen. Pract.; M.D.; In practice prior to the Act of 1815; formerly Apoth. to the Bristol Infirmary; Surg. To the Hundred of Stow, and the Dorcas Society; Mem. Of the Council of the Prov. Med. and Surg. Association, and of the Nat. Instit.; Author of 'The Enemy of Empiricism', and of a 'Compendium of Medical Practice'; contributor of numerous papers to the *Lancet, Provin. Med and Surg. Journal* and *Dublin Med. Press* on Medicine, Surgery and Midwifery, on Medical Reform, and the New Poor Law.

FERNELEY, Charles, Denton, near Grantham, Lincolnshire-Gen. Pract.; M.R.C.S. 1833; Med. Officer to Grantham Union. Author of 'Lectures on Nutrition of Plants'. Contributed to *Med. Gaz.* a paper 'On certain Medical Laws which obtain in the Animal Economy', Jan. 1840.

MOTT, William Hadley, Kemp Town, Brighton-Surgeon; in practice prior to the Act of 1815; formerly Surgeon in the Army.

Selected entries from the *Provincial Medical Directory* (1847), London: John Churchill (pp. 20, 23, 98, 200) quoted in Webster, 2001 (p. 50).

1 What strikes you about the use of the term 'general practitioner' in these entries?
2 What are the features of those who give themselves this designation?
3 What range of activities do these entrants also undertake?
4 What role do publications play?

Feedback

1 Some doctors use the term 'general practitioner', but not all of them. Some who seem to be general practitioners in the modern use of the term do not call themselves by this name. It is clear that this is not yet a professional term in universal use.
2 They are very diverse in the activities that they undertake. Many stress that they were in practice prior to the 1815 Act.
3 They undertake a wide range of activities – surgeon to the Great Western Railway, for example, or public vaccinator.

4 Having published something, of whatever type, is clearly seen as a professional advantage and something that supports professional status. See the entry for James Bedingfield of Stowmarket.

Formal credentials remained very confusing. Until the Medical Act of 1858, between fifteen and twenty bodies could offer different qualifications. This was the period of the medical reform movement. There were attacks by rank-and-file practitioners on the London Royal Colleges and medical elites, and in 1832 a separate professional organization representing general practitioners was founded, the Provincial Medical and Surgical Association, which later became the British Medical Association. One of the leading lights of this campaign was the radical surgeon and Member of Parliament Thomas Wakley, who was editor of the medical journal the Lancet. In its early years, the journal was a radical force, waging war against the incompetence of the medical elite.

Exercise 4.2

Read the following extract from the Lancet published in 1827/8. It comments on an operation that had been carried out by the nephew of Sir Astley Cooper, a leading London surgeon. Then answer the questions that follow.

'Guy's Hospital

THE OPERATION OF LITHOTOMY BY MR BRANSBY COOPER, WHICH LASTED NEARLY ONE HOUR!!

…It will, doubtless, be useful to the country 'draff' [ordinary people who live in the country] to learn how things are managed by one of the privileged order – a Hospital surgeon – nephew and surgeon, and surgeon because he is a 'nephew'.

The performance of this tragedy was nearly as follows [there followed a dramatic eye witness account of the bungled operation by Cooper, after which the patient died; another patient ran away from the hospital]

> …When Cooper's *nevey* cut for stone,
> His toils were long and heavy;
> This patient quicker parts [internal organs] has shown,
> He *soon cut* Cooper's *nevey*.

…Such are the men who style themselves the heads of the profession! Such is the race of hospital apprentices, *neveys* [nephews], and noodles [derogatory term for someone without knowledge] who insolently domineer over the great body of the profession! What, it has been asked, must the priests have been in a country, where the god was a monkey! If such men were at the head of the profession, who could be at its tail? The truth is, we repeat, that the highest degree of professional knowledge and skill, as well as the greatest amount of intelligence and activity, is to be found among that enlightened, though hitherto degraded class, which has been stigmatised by the corrupt few, as a *subordinate* department of the profession. In conclusion, we earnestly impress it as a rule of conduct, subject to a few, and very few exceptions, on all who value the health and lives of those who are near and dear to them: "*So long as the present corrupt system of patronage continues* avoid the men who style themselves the heads of the profession; above all, avoid the metropolitan hospital physicians and surgeons".'

1 What does the writer (Wakley) object to about this operation?
2 What does he criticize about the way in which the profession is organized?
3 What do you think about the tone and language of the extract?

Feedback

1 The operation was unnecessarily lengthy (and thus very painful in the absence of anaesthesia); it was carried out incompetently; it was carried out by the nephew of the great surgeon and thus nepotism had been involved.
2 The writer criticizes the system of London based hospital dominated physicians and surgeons who operate an apprentice system. He emphasizes that the greatest degree of training and competence in the medical profession is to be found outside London, and is located in the qualified general or primary care practitioners who operate outside the corrupt London system.
3 The tone is bold and uninhibited. It is unlike the language one would expect in a medical journal today, but it represents the radicalism of the emergent general practitioner and his challenge to orthodox medicine.

Specialists and generalists

The historian Jeanne Peterson has argued that another period of professional unification and consolidation came between the 1858 Act and a further Amendment Act in 1886 (Peterson, 1978). The bulk of this Act dealt with medical licensing in the colonies, but it also required that the examination of all three main branches of medicine – medicine, surgery and midwifery – be compulsory. Specialisms in medicine multiplied in the last half of the century and the idea of a laboratory-based training slowly spread in England after it had become the norm in Germany and the United States. In Germany, research became an essential component of medicine and a strong biomedical clinical influence was brought to bear. The 1910 Flexner Report proposed that all American medical education be based on the German model. This ideal was already an important influence, for example, on the Johns Hopkins School of Medicine, founded in Baltimore in 1889. In Britain, there was reluctance to embrace the emphasis on research and full-time academic appointments did not develop in the London medical schools until after the First World War.

Professional success continued to be linked to social status and family connections, and underpinned the distinction between consultant and general practitioner (GP). This divide was sharpened in British medicine after the 1911 National Health Insurance Act (discussed in more detail in Chapter 9). A GP service became available to manual workers and the principle of GP referral to hospital led to a much sharper distinction between the consultant-based hospital service and general practitioners. Qualified medical practice remained a male preserve until the 1860s and the first women entrants in Britain and the US had to follow a path of separate development, in separate medical schools and even hospitals. Women practitioners later tended to be concentrated in specialities relating to women and children or in lower status options such as the School Medical Service. The major aspects of the gendered division of labour in health care are discussed below.

Public health professionals

During this period, and slightly later than the rise of general practice, came the establishment of a formal public health profession. There were different views of how a public health workforce might operate. In the eighteenth century in the absolutist European states, the concept of medical police (the idea promoted in European authoritarian states from the eighteenth century to promote state control in the medical sphere through systems of inspection and enforcement through the criminal law) had been common. This idea was promoted by the physician Johann Peter Frank from 1779 to assert the role of the state in the medical sphere. His system of state-administered preventive and curative medicine had widespread influence in Europe. The policing model of public health was to remain influential in Britain. For example, in the 1830s the Factory Inspectorate was established and in the 1850s, building on the ideas promoted by John Simon, Medical Officers of Health were established who had compulsory powers under the criminal law. There was also a more radical European model. Concepts of social medicine were introduced in France in the 1830s and disseminated more widely in Europe. The notion of health care as a democratic right emerged in the German medical reform movement in the revolutions of 1848–1849. These ideas were to re-emerge in the 1930s and 1940s.

In practice, the role of the Medical Officer of Health, which developed in the UK in the second half of the nineteenth century, was a less radical, but no less significant one. These officials were at first attached to temporary Boards of Health in periods of epidemic crisis, before becoming compulsory in London districts in 1855 and in all local government areas in the 1870s. Despite their importance at the local level and the formal recognition in 1886 of the Diploma in Public Health as their professional qualification, the Medical Officer of Health remained the Cinderella of the medical profession (Porter, 1991). Yet their responsibilities were wide and included the removal of nuisances, the regulation of overcrowded lodging houses, building standards, the condition of bakeries, dairies and slaughter-houses. From 1889 they enforced prevention of infectious diseases through notification and isolation and by the turn of the century they increasingly supervised local services such as health visiting, thus prefiguring their later role running a wider range of services in the inter-war years (discussed in more detail in Chapter 11).

Exercise 4.3

The following extract comes from a letter written by one of the most famous Medical Officers of Health of this period. For four years (1884–1888), Arthur Newsholme was a part-time Medical Officer of Health in Clapham in London where he divided his time between public health work and general practice. Then for twenty years (1888–1908) he was full-time Medical Officer of Health in Brighton, where he helped to build a model public health programme. His career as a public health administrator and epidemiologist there shows the influence public health officials could have at the local level. As Medical Officer of the Local Government Board from 1908, he was a central government civil servant, the head of public health, at a time when the Liberal welfare initiatives (see Chapter 10) were being passed. After his retirement in 1919, he remained influential on both sides of the Atlantic; in the United States he was on the board of the newly created Johns Hopkins School of Hygiene and Public Health (Eyler, 1997).

The extract shows how Newsholme dealt with the results of local research, which showed that tuberculosis was passed from one infected person to another. Compulsory notification was not practical and so he began the process of securing voluntary notification of cases of tuberculosis.

Read the extract from the letter he sent to local medical practitioners and then answer the questions that follow.

'I beg therefore to invite you to cooperate with me in notifying cases of Phthisis [tuberculosis] occurring in your practice, where in your opinion public good can be achieved by such notification. I may remind you that even though in the individual case under your care no further precautions and no sanitary improvements are required, the official knowledge of your case may direct my attention to "infected areas" and possibly be the means of facilitating important sanitary reforms.

There will, I need hardly say, be no official interference, as the result of the notification, with your patient, either at home or in connection with his occupation, the steps taken being confined to a sanitary inspection of the house and giving a copy of the card to the patient or responsible relative.'

1 What reasons does Newsholme give for seeking the cooperation of local general practitioners?
2 How does he differentiate between the work of a public health doctor and that of a primary health doctor?

Feedback

1 Newsholme wants cooperation in notification so as to secure the public good and to help with sanitary improvement. He wants to identify infected areas rather than infected individuals so that improvements to the overall environment can be initiated.
2 The work of a public health doctor will deal with infected areas, not with the treatment of individual patients. Newsholme stresses that there will be no official interference with the patient in his home or in his occupation. He stresses the separation between prevention and treatment and between public and private health care. Newsholme is concerned to reassure the general practitioner that his arena of medicine will not be taken over by the public health official. His letter stresses the difference between the interest of the general practitioner, which is confined to the individual patient, and that of the public health doctor, which is concerned with the population as a whole and in preventing further infection through sanitary improvements.

This British model of public health personnel did not apply in all countries. In the United States, as historian Elizabeth Fee has shown, other professional groups were active and interested and often more willing to accept salaried employment. Professional competition between sanitary engineers and doctors became intense in the early years of the twentieth century. Many doctors preferred private practice where the financial rewards were greater (Fee, 1991).

Lay care and other emergent professions

The extension of medical power did not mark the end of older traditions of folk medicine and self-medication. During most of the period with which this book deals, much medicine was self-prescribed and self-administered. The free dispensaries, poor law infirmaries and outpatient departments of the voluntary hospitals provided a limited form of orthodox medical care. But the bulk of poor people dealt with everyday ailments themselves.

In its simplest form, folk medicine was based on herbs, flowers and roots that could easily be grown or gathered in a rural setting and which appeared in standard herbals that were published well into the nineteenth century. Country traditions were also carried over into the urban setting. The character of Old Alice in *Mary Barton* (1848), Mrs Gaskell's novel of industrial life, illustrates this. Alice lives in a cellar in Manchester but her skills derive from a preindustrial era:

> She had been out all day in the fields, gathering wild herbs for drinks and medicine, for in addition to her invaluable qualities as a sick nurse and her worldly occupation as a washerwoman, she added a considerable knowledge of hedge and field simples.

The role of pharmacists in lay medical care was also considerable. Pharmacists, like doctors, were also professionalizing. In England, they achieved a form of professional status between the formation of the Pharmaceutical Society in 1841 to the passing of a Pharmacy Act in 1868. These developments established a regulated system of education for 'pharmaceutical chemists' and a schedule of drugs (including the great standby, opium, which is discussed in greater detail in Chapter 7) that only they could dispense. But the conflict between professional status and trade was not entirely solved. The local corner pharmacist had a mainly working and lower middle class clientele. He combined prescribing over the counter with often making up family recipes that were brought in.

Exercise 4.4

The following is from an interview with a pharmacist who worked in the north of England remembering how customers used his shop. Read the extract from the interview and then answer the questions that follow.

'Pharmacist:　We were the first filter as it were … we had to do a bit of diagnosing in our own way and be responsible for it.

Interviewer:　Would they for example bring children in and [ask] "What is the matter?"

Pharmacist:　Oh my goodness yes.

Interviewer:　What sort of things would be the matter with them?

Pharmacist:　It might be just nettle rash, it might be measles – very often it was measles and teething trouble, a little feverish, constipation or something like that, the usual childish ailments but we had to be very, very careful in case there was little yellow spots behind the throat and then write to the doctor …'

Interviewer:　You didn't charge for advice?

Pharmacist:　Oh dear no. Everything had to be inexpensive …'

(Roberts, 1980, p. 45)

1 What role is the pharmacist carrying out?

2 What is the relationship between the pharmacist and the doctor?

3 Does anything strike you about the role of the pharmacist here in relation to the current role of the occupation in your country?

Feedback

1 The pharmacist is acting as a primary health care practitioner. His role is wider than simply that of dispensing drugs, for he is diagnosing and treating patients as well.

2 The pharmacist is careful not to overstep the boundaries with regular medical practice. If the illness seems likely to be serious, then the case is referred to a doctor.

3 In the UK, pharmacy has re-emerged as part of primary health care and the role of the pharmacist as a public health practitioner has also been emphasized in recent years. Pharmacists have been used, for example, to distribute nicotine replacement therapy to smokers and for needle exchange and maintenance medication for drug addicts. The pharmacist's shop is also seen as a place where advice on health matters can be obtained. In your country this may be different. The pharmacist may be in competition with the local general practitioners, or there may not be any general practitioners. Maybe general practice is not a standard profession there or they may be unavailable or inaccessible. In the latter case, the pharmacist may play the role of primary care provider as the occupation does in many low-income countries.

Pharmacy was also part of a strong commercial tendency. There was an increased sale of patent medicines towards the end of the nineteenth century and newspaper advertising expanded. The advertising expenditure of pharmaceutical entrepreneurs in the UK such as Thomas Beecham and Thomas Holloway increased rapidly towards the end of the nineteenth century. There were many abuses of patent medicine sale and advertisement. Leading public figures were quoted as endorsing products they had probably never heard of and it was common to state that a medicine did not contain opium when it did. These abuses were attacked in campaigns both in the UK and in the United States promoted by the medical and pharmaceutical professions at the turn of the nineteenth and twentieth centuries.

The gendered division of health labour: Nursing, midwifery and health visiting

The establishment of professional medical organizations had further implications for women's role in health care. It led to the marginalization of specifically female healers and to the establishment of a number of health care professions such as nursing, midwifery and health visiting that were subordinate to male medical practice. In this section of the chapter, we look at how these professions developed and how they established their role in part by denigrating the role of practitioners who had preceded them.

Nursing

At first sight, the history of nursing seems to exemplify the power of medical reform and a story of progress in the nineteenth century. In his novel *Martin Chuzzlewit*, Charles Dickens portrayed pre-reform nursing as a low-grade occupation ripe for reform. His characters Sarah Gamp and Betsy Prig were down at heel, drunken and elderly. However, this picture can be too readily accepted and the following exercise is intended to help you think about nursing in the nineteenth century more critically.

Exercise 4.5

The following quotation describes Sally Dunkirk, a female practitioner in Yorkshire in the 1860s. Read the extract and then answer the questions that follow.

> 'Any bad case of fever, or lunacy, of exceptional emergency, was a call for Sally's services. In such cases she became general, and house maid, doctor and nurse, friend and physician all in one ... A most useful woman was she for the times in which she lived ... If her treatment failed to restore the patient to normal health it was a case forthwith to be sent to a lunatic asylum. Her fees were never much more than a liberal supply of home-brewed beer, unrestricted stock of good "bacca" [tobacco] and the indispensable long clay pipe, with a good "table" [provision of ample food supplies], and implicit obedience to her orders.'
>
> (quoted in Marland, 1987, p. 219)

1 What strikes you about the sort of care that Sally is providing? What does it comprise?
2 How does she relate to orthodox medical practice?
3 How does this account of a female practitioner compare with the description given by Dickens?

Feedback

1 Sally is providing medical and nursing care rolled into one, but she is also providing household services as well, such as a home help might have provided in later times.
2 Her work seems to be distinct from medical practice. She will send cases to a lunatic asylum if they are disordered, but otherwise there is no mention of liaison with doctors.
3 Some of the elements of this description tally with the picture given by Dickens: Sally is paid in drink and tobacco and given food and lodging. But the emphasis in this description is entirely different and is not made into a case for reform. Sally is seen as an independent practitioner whose norms are acceptable to the community in which she operates.

So you might conclude that some elements of the case for reform need to be questioned. Nursing as a Christian duty was traditionally associated with the female role. Reforming work was initiated by religious sisterhoods and carried further by the work of Florence Nightingale in the Crimean War in the 1850s. Poor hospital care of the troops created a national scandal in the press (this was the first military venture reported by war correspondents). Nightingale used her social connections with the Secretary of War, Sidney Herbert, to obtain an appointment to lead a party of nurses to the Crimea. The real impact of her work there is controversial; improvements to the mortality rates in the military hospital at Scutari appear not to have been associated with nursing. However, the image of Nightingale, the caring nurse, the 'Lady with the Lamp' became an important patriotic symbol in a war marked by military and planning blunders. On her return to Britain, Nightingale took advantage of her celebrity to publicize her ideas on military medicine and sanitation. The work of the Nightingale School, attached to St. Thomas' Hospital in London in 1861, was important in establishing nursing as a professional occupation suitable for middle- and upper-class women. Florence Nightingale is remembered as the key figure in the transition of nursing from a low-status occupation to a skilled profession. Her *Notes on Nursing*, first published in 1859 and revised several times, was instrumental in setting out the essential aspects of the theory and practice of nursing.

Exercise 4.6

The following are extracts from sections written about nursing by Florence Nightingale for the *Encyclopaedia Britannica* in 1893. Read through the extracts and then answer the questions that follow.

'Nursing is, above all, a progressive calling. Year by year nurses have to learn new and improved methods, as medicine and surgery and hygiene improve ... Further, year by year, nursing needs to be more and more of a moral calling.

...A really good nurse must need be of the highest class of character. It need hardly be said that she must be (1) Chaste, in the sense of the Sermon on the Mount ... it is the only case, queens not excepted, where a woman is really in charge of men. And a really good trained ward 'sister' can keep order in a men's ward better than a military ward master or sergeant. (2) Sober, in spirit as well as in drink ... (3) Honest, not accepting the most trifling fee or bribe from patients or friends. (4) Truthful ... (5) Trustworthy, to carry out directions intelligently and perfectly, unseen as well as seen, 'to the Lord' as well as unto men-no mere eye service; (6) Punctual to a second and orderly to a hair ... (7) Quiet, yet quick ... gentle without slowness; discreet without self importance; no gossip; (8) Cheerful, hopeful ... (9) Cleanly to the point of exquisiteness, both for the patient's sake and her own; neat and ready; (10) Thinking of her patient and not of herself ... she must have a rule of thought; and this the physician or surgeon has to give her in his directions; which her training must have fitted her to obey intelligently, using discretion ... Half the battle of nursing is to relieve your sick from having to think for themselves at all-least of all for their own nursing.'

1 What are the main characteristics of a good nurse?
2 How does the role of the nurse compare with that of the doctor?
3 What is the relationship of the nurse and the patient?
4 How does this view of nursing compare with that practised by Sally Dunkirk in Exercise 4.5?

Feedback

1 The main characteristics of a good nurse are partly moral – chastity, honesty, selflessness – and also physical, what were thought of at the time as 'female' characteristics such as cleanliness and quietness.

2 The nurse has to keep up to date to be able to serve medicine and hygiene. She is also the agent of the doctor, able to carry out his orders.

3 The nurse commends the patient, in particular on the men's ward but also in carrying out what is seen as best for the patient and not allowing him or her to speak or think for him or herself.

4 This is a very different view of nursing. The nurse is not an independent practitioner, but is subordinate to doctors. The moral aspect of her professional identity is important. She does not drink and has to be chaste. Sally Dunkirk was part of the community in which she lived, while Nightingale's view of nursing seems to be an institutional one. There is a definite hierarchy in which the patient is at the bottom of the pile, below both doctor and nurse.

Nineteenth-century nursing reform was partly driven by a desire for efficiency in the public sphere but also confirmed the gender divide by stressing female subordination to the male medical hierarchy. Historians have commented that many of the changes concerned with Nightingale nurses, with respect to skills, social background and ethos, would have happened anyway because they met the needs of hospital doctors. And some areas of nursing, for example in the Poor Law, remained almost untouched by the Nightingale improvements. Perhaps in the words of the historian F.B. Smith (1982), 'Miss Nightingale served the cause of nursing less than it served her'.

Midwifery

Midwifery was another area where the needs of medical men also began to dominate. In the seventeenth century, most babies were delivered by women. But in the eighteenth century, more men came into this area of practice, aided by technological innovation, the midwifery forceps, which were not available to midwives in their practice. Soon the stereotype of 'ignorant midwives' was commonplace, much as the image of drunken old hags had tainted untrained nurses. By the middle of the nineteenth century, midwives were virtually confined to attendance on the poor, combining help at childbirth with general work such as washing and cleaning.

Moves by women of professional status to enter medicine had their impact on midwifery as well as on medicine and nursing. The emergence of a class of highly educated and vocal midwives as a professionalizing pressure group led to efforts in the last three decades of the nineteenth century to bring about training and control. The battle in the UK was between medical pressure groups seeking legislation to control midwives in their own interests, and the middle-class section of midwifery seeking independent professional status. The 1902 Midwives Act was a compromise. It prohibited unqualified practice but placed midwifery in a disadvantaged position in the gendered division of labour. The ruling Central Midwives Board had a medical majority and supervision at the local level was by the Medical Officer of Health. The immediate impact on unqualified practice was muted, for women in 'bona fide practice' were allowed to continue their work.

Exercise 4.7

The two images below are from the history of midwifery. In picture A on the left, which dates from the late eighteenth century, the midwife is portrayed as half male and half female, half surgeon and half midwife. In picture B on the right, which is by T. Rowlandson (1811), a midwife is shown going to attend a labour in the middle of the night.

Look at the pictures and then answer the questions that follow.

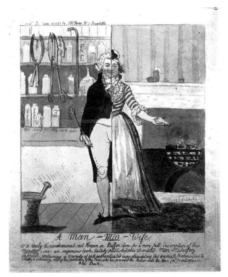 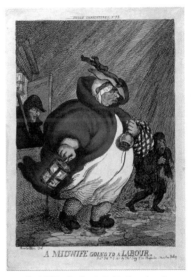

Figure 4.1 A (left): Samuel William Fores, 'Man-midwifery dissected', 1793. B (right): T. Rowlandson, A midwife going to a labour, 1811

Credit: Wellcome Library, London

1 What does the portrayal of the man midwife in picture A imply? What does this creature say about the nature of midwifery?
2 What do you notice about the portrayal of the midwife in picture B? What does it imply about the state of midwifery?

Feedback

1 The picture implies that the professional is neither one thing nor the other. The midwife is half-man and half-woman and the picture implies that this is unnatural. Note in the background on the male side of the picture the various implements that the male surgeons were able to use – the forceps and other instruments that gave men control over childbirth and that were not available to female midwives in their practice.
2 The midwife is fat and rather unkempt. She is carrying a lantern and what looks like a bottle of alcohol. The portrayal is part of the denigration of female midwifery, which was well in train by the first half of the nineteenth century. This is an unsympathetic portrayal of possibly unqualified practice. We would need to assess its value

as evidence against other sources that testify to the role of such practitioners in the lives of the poor.

Health visiting

The Medical Officers of Health also came to take charge of another group of women health workers. These were the health visitors who became part of the local government based public health service in the UK at the time of the First World War.

Volunteer visiting of the poor had a long history but this became more marked from about the 1860s. In 1862, the Ladies' section of the Manchester and Salford Sanitary Association began to spread health information among the poor of the community. Visiting nurses moved rapidly to other areas, promoting the care and welfare of children at home. Some writers specifically drew the contrast between male public health labour, which dealt with sanitation and engineering, and that suitable for women.

The main development at the end of the nineteenth century was that such visitors were more likely to have a trained background. Formal health visiting schemes expanded in the early years of the twentieth century and ultimately came under the control of Medical Officers of Health. By 1918, health visitor numbers had reached a thousand and in 1919 uniform training requirements had been laid down. Their position was ambiguous in that they were expected to befriend and gently influence, but also to monitor and report. There has been disagreement between historians about the role of health visiting and its impact. Jane Lewis (1980) has pointed to the limited nature of the services on offer, which focused only on advice and not on treatment, because of the focus on individual self-help and responsibility. Deborah Dwork (1987), however, argues that their work led to a significant downturn in the infant mortality rate. Lara Marks (1996) has also pointed to the shift in expectations and ethos round such services in London in the inter-war years. Services became more inclusive and less patronizing and the relationship between health visitors and mothers more equal.

Summary

We have seen how different health professions established themselves during this period. The divide between hospital and primary health care services underpinned the division between consultant and general practitioner. Public health also developed its own professional workforce, in part structured round a gendered division of labour with male medical public health professionals directing a female workforce of midwives and health visitors. But for many 'health consumers' lay care remained common along with self-medication. The role of the pharmacist remained important as a semi-professional source of advice and a meeting point for lay and professional involvement in health care. In the next chapter, we explore the work of health professionals over a similar period, but in a different context: when European colonists took Western medicine to the 'tropical' world.

References and further reading

Berridge V (1990) Health and medicine, in Thompson FML (ed) *The Cambridge Social History of Britain, 1750–1950: Vol. 3. Social agencies and institutions.* Cambridge: Cambridge University Press.

Dickens C (2004) *Martin Chuzzlewit.* London: Penguin.

Digby A (1999) *The Evolution of British General Practice, 1850–1948*. Oxford: Oxford University Press.

Dingwall R, Rafferty AM and Webster C (1988) *An Introduction to the Social History of Nursing*. London: Routledge.

Dwork D (1987) *War is Good for Babies and Other Young Children: A History of the Infant and Child Welfare Movement in Britain, 1898–1918*. London: Tavistock.

Eyler J (1997) *Sir Arthur Newsholme and State Medicine, 1885–1935*. Cambridge: Cambridge University Press.

Fee E (1991) Designing schools of public health for the United States, in Fee E and Acheson R (eds) *A History of Education in Public Health: Health that Mocks the Doctors' Rules*, pp. 155–94. Oxford: Oxford Medical Publications.

Fee E and Acheson R (eds) (1991) *A History of Education in Public Health: Health that Mocks the Doctors' Rules*. Oxford: Oxford Medical Publications.

Gaskell Mrs E (1848/1970) *Mary Barton*. London: Penguin.

Lewis J (1980) *The Politics of Motherhood: Child and Maternal Welfare in England, 1900–1939*. London: Croom Helm.

Loudon I (1987) *Medical Care and the General Practitioner, 1750–1850*. Oxford: Clarendon Press.

Marks L (1996) *Metropolitan Maternity: Maternal and Infant Welfare Services in Early Twentieth Century London*. Amsterdam: Rodopi.

Marland H (1987) *Medicine and Society in Wakefield and Huddersfield, 1780–1870*. Cambridge: Cambridge University Press.

Peterson J (1978) *The Medical Profession in mid Victorian London*. Berkeley, CA: University of California Press.

Porter D (1991) Stratification and its discontents: Professionalization and conflict in the British public health service, in Fee E and Acheson R (eds) *A History of Education in Public Health: Health that Mocks the Doctors' Rules*, pp. 83–113. Oxford: Oxford Medical Publications.

Roberts E (1980) Oral history investigations of disease and its management by the Lancashire working class, 1890–1939, in Pickstone J (ed) *Health, Disease and Medicine in Lancashire, 1750–1850*. Occasional Publication No. 2. Manchester: UMIST.

Smith FB (1982) *Florence Nightingale: Reputation and Power*. London: Croom Helm.

Webster C (2001) *Caring for Health: History and Diversity* (3rd edn). Buckingham: Open University Press.

5 | Tropical medicine

John Manton

Overview

In this chapter, we explore the reasons for the emergence of tropical medicine as a distinct medical specialism in the years up to 1945. We will discover how medical specialists and public health administrators worked to reconcile new approaches to the management of vector-borne diseases with colonial and national concerns over tropical agricultural productivity. To explain this process, we examine the roots and changing understandings of poverty in tropical latitudes, and subsequent public health responses.

Learning objectives

After working through this chapter, you will be able to:

- describe the relations between the emergence of tropical medicine and the exercise of imperial power
- use primary sources to identify and explain some of the factors and problems shaping public health in tropical and semi-tropical colonies of European powers
- analyse the historical relation between global relations of inequality and the problems addressed by tropical medicine

Key terms

Anopheles mosquitoes The species of mosquito that transmits the malaria parasite.

Colonial (in medicine) Relating to medical planning, programmes or institutions specific to a given colonial territory.

Disease control A reduction in the rate of transmission of endemic or epidemic disease, using a systematic and planned approach.

Eugenics The science of human heredity informed by Darwinian evolutionary theory. This was linked in the early twentieth century to racial improvement and the prevention of degeneration through a variety of different strategies. 'Negative eugenics' proposed strategies such as sterilization. 'Positive eugenics' promoted welfare policies and interventions to improve the quality of the population.

Hookworm A nematode (roundworm) intestinal parasite of humans. Infection is through direct contact with contaminated soil. Heavy infection can cause anaemia and weight loss, and is associated with developmental problems in children.

Imperial (in medicine) Relating to empire-wide or imperial metropolitan (e.g. London, Paris) medical planning, institutions, practice or programmes.

Leprosy A chronic disease of bacillary origin, primarily affecting the skin, peripheral nerves and mucosa. It has an exceptionally long incubation period (c. 5 years) and is only mildly infectious. It is curable, and early treatment can prevent disability and disfigurement. Historically, social stigma has strongly affected the control and management of leprosy.

Racial hygiene Science originating in nineteenth-century Germany that warned of the effects of social policies and medical care which helped the weak and unfit to survive. Linked with theories of evolution and heredity and considered the health of the race as a whole as well as that of the individual. This was important in many countries but in particular in Germany.

Sleeping sickness Or human African trypanosomiasis, is a protozoan disease transmitted by the tsetse fly. It is found in sub-Saharan Africa, and can affect the central nervous system, and it is fatal unless treated.

Social hygiene Another branch of social biology that favoured rather than opposed preventive medicine. Social hygiene aimed to analyse the effect of social conditions on health and mortality. Term used extensively in the inter-war years, for example in the naming of the London School of Hygiene and Tropical Medicine.

Vector-borne disease A disease in which the pathogen (e.g. virus or bacteria) is transmitted to humans or mammals by a living carrier or *vector*, such as mosquitoes, ticks or flies.

Introduction

Tropical medicine emerged as a distinct medical specialism towards the close of the nineteenth century. For the first half of the twentieth century, this specialism consisted of a specific set of techniques applied to the management of a limited range of infectious diseases, largely of vector-borne parasitic origin. It was intimately bound to issues of hygiene, labour control and public order experienced in European colonial governance in Africa and Asia, and in the drive to exploit natural resources in Latin America. In this chapter, we examine the problems tropical medicine sought to solve, and the social and ideological tensions that beset medical practice in tropical climatic conditions and in the colonial world.

It is important to understand that the term 'tropical' only loosely applies in relating health to climate. The period from the early 1870s to 1945 witnessed rapid developments in microbiology, chemotherapy and parasitology. This period also saw competitive militarization, rapid European imperial expansion and commodity-driven industrialization. This industrialization relied increasingly on the close control of labour and agricultural production in Latin America, Africa and Asia. The new potential for field scientific research offered by territorial and institutional expansion saw the development of schools of tropical medicine across Europe at the turn of the twentieth century. All of these processes went hand-in-hand with ecological and social disruption arising from early colonial ventures in plantation agriculture and the harvesting of forest produce, as well as with urbanization in the more globally integrated economies of Latin America and South Asia.

LIVERPOOL JOHN MOORES UNIVERSITY
LEARNING SERVICES

At the same time, critical perspectives on colonial health and welfare, voiced by medical workers and missionaries, among other critics of imperialism, formed an important part of the tropical medical vision. Such critics sought always to contextualize 'tropical medicine' in relation to emerging discourses on social medicine and public health examined in Chapter 10 of this book.

Exercise 5.1

Thinking about the country in which you live, give examples of *three* of the major diseases associated with poverty. For each example, decide whether the cause is primarily social, environmental, dietary or infectious. Give a reason for your decision.

Feedback

You will have given different examples depending on where you live. As we saw in Chapters 2 and 3, during the nineteenth century, cholera, typhus and dietary deficiencies were common expressions of the effect of poverty on health across much of the industrial world, including Britain.

You may have chosen obesity as one of the major diseases associated with poverty today. The 'epidemic of obesity' and the increased prevalence of Type 2 diabetes are nowadays associated with poverty across an ever-increasing geographic domain, comprising countries in the developing and developed world.

Other diseases, especially vector-borne infections such as malaria, yellow fever and dengue fever, and mycobacterial infections such as leprosy and tuberculosis – commonly associated with poor sanitary conditions and, apart from tuberculosis, with tropical climates – have all existed at some point over the past millennium in zones currently described as semi-tropical and temperate (e.g. Dobson, 1980, who outlines the epidemiology of malaria in southern England).

The increase of cancers and depression in the developing world reflect a complex mix of factors, which are not easy to distinguish. The changing global profile of tobacco use, and its relation to marketing and regulation, is a case in point.

The emergence of the tropics

The evolution of a distinctive 'tropical medicine' relied on differentiating tropical from temperate geographical zones. However, it also relied on separating the tropics as objects of study from the (European) zones in which scientific knowledge was produced and debated. In addition, the forms of medicine and public health practised at 'tropical' latitudes, irrespective of actual climate and topography, were in many cases linked by colonial experience. Whether in the hill stations of India, the Kenya Highlands, the West African Gold Coast or colonial Calcutta, the relations between health worker and general public owed more to colonial than to climatic conditions.

The history of European exploration from the fifteenth century, and the growth of mercantile empires in the seventeenth and eighteenth centuries gave rise to a need to distinguish and understand ecological zones and exotic societies. The development of cartography, geography, taxonomy and the sciences of classification in the eighteenth and nineteenth centuries equipped Europeans with a language with which they could describe this newly encountered global human and biological variety and difference. Concerns with scientific enlightenment and economic development, emerging in the towns, gardens, factories and farms of late-Georgian Britain (*c.* 1770 to 1830), became central to the management of tropical agriculture in South Asia and the Caribbean (Drayton, 2000).

Nineteenth-century observations of the tropics were heavily indebted to the work of the German geographer Alexander von Humboldt, whose travels in Latin America at the beginning of the nineteenth century did much to popularize the connection between tropical climatic zones and fertile plant life (Stepan, 2006). Humboldt was less immediately concerned with animal and human life, but the mid nineteenth century popularization of metaphors of selection and extinction seen, for example, in Charles Darwin's *Origin of the Species*, gave rise to ideological links, discussed in Chapter 10, between place, population health and race, in disciplines such as social and racial hygiene, and eugenics.

Specific concerns arose with the increasing migration of Europeans to new imperial territories. For much of the nineteenth century, European residence in the tropics was confined to small trading garrisons. Even in India, the British East India Company managed British trading and military concerns in the subcontinent largely through Indian agency until the Crown assumed control of the government of India in the wake of the Indian Rebellion of 1857. As the administrative remit of Empire grew, and the economic and strategic value of colonization became widely accepted among European powers, so did concerns with the health and survival of Europeans quartered among colonial subjects in the cities and provinces of British, French, Belgian, Dutch and German empires.

Before the technical and intellectual developments in microbiology and bacteriology that underpinned germ theory, and new models of disease causation proposed by scientists such as Louis Pasteur and Robert Koch (explored in Chapter 2), the management of European health in the tropics was largely spatial. The main angles of attack on poorly understood diseases were sanitary and exclusionary. In garrisons, better hygiene and a reduction in overcrowding in the middle years of the nineteenth century were key to improved military mortality in tropical conditions (Curtin, 1989).

The reputation of modern medicine and medical practitioners was by no means established. While the impact of biomedicine had begun to take root in India in the second half of the twentieth century, for most of Africa beyond the garrison, the epidemiological landscape remained largely a mystery. Beyond slave ports and strategic enclaves, the health impact of colonial social upheaval on societies in Africa, Asia and Australasia was also poorly understood.

In terms of disease causation, it was not until 1873 that a bacterial pathogen was first proposed for a disease. The disease was leprosy, and the pathogen was identified by Armauer Hansen, a Norwegian (Norway had a long-standing leprosy problem, strongly associated with extreme poverty). The infectiousness of leprosy continued to be debated well into the middle of the twentieth century. Thus, social arrangements seen as encouraging overcrowding and poor sanitation, and dietary factors such as poor nutrition and overreliance on specific food items (notably fish!) continued to arouse the suspicion of public health officials from the late nineteenth century until after the Second World War.

Exercise 5.2

Maps are a useful way of representing data on all manner of measurable indicators, especially when it comes to visualizing distribution. Given strong datasets, maps enable us to query anomalies in distribution, to identify shortcomings in data collection, as well as

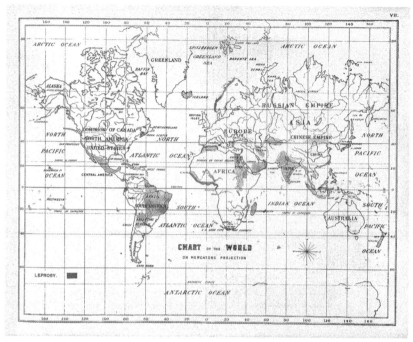

Figure 5.1 Map of the world showing distribution of Leprosy

Source: Felkin (1889)

Credit: Wellcome Library, London

generate new avenues of investigation. In the map below, taken from the 1889 publication *On the Geographical Distribution of Some Tropical Diseases, and their Relation to Physical Phenomena*, by R.W. Felkin, an Edinburgh-based lecturer on diseases of the tropics and climatology, the global distribution of leprosy is shown by the shaded areas. Note the shading of Iceland, coastal Norway and Nova Scotia alongside zones more commonly associated with the practice of tropical medicine, and then answer the questions that follow.

1 Apart from the presumed prevalence of leprosy, what factors do you think might unify the shaded areas on the map?
2 Why is Africa largely unshaded? (Note the areas of Africa that *are* shaded.)
3 What do you think maps add to our understanding of disease distribution? In what ways might they be counter-productive?

Feedback

1 While no single feature unites all of the shaded areas on the map, widespread poverty in a given society (mid nineteenth century Iceland, Norway and Nova Scotia share this experience with much of India and large areas of post-slavery Brazil) *or* recent experience of massive social upheaval (as in Japan and New Zealand) indicate societal factors that might increase susceptibility to disease in a population.
2 At the time of compilation of this map, published in 1889, the areas shaded in Africa – the Maghreb, coastal West Africa south of the Sahel, the South African Cape and its

hinterland, Madagascar and coastal Tanganyika, and the Nile Basin – comprised the extent of European exploitation of labour and land to date.

3 In reading maps we need to be aware of potential gaps in the data. If an area represented on the map is poorly represented in a dataset, this will need to be reflected in the context in which we read the map. Beyond this, the history of cartography understands mapping as a political process. In using maps as a historical source, we must remember to engage in a critical reading of these, as of any other source. It may well be the case, for instance, that readers of Felkin's 1889 volume would assume inland Africa and Australia to be data-free zones, and would not expect to read knowledge of such areas in any world map!

The development of 'tropical medicine'

At the same time as sanitary interventions improved health among Europeans in the tropics, the rapid development in microbiology in Europe shed light on models of disease transmission in some of the major illnesses we now know to be vector-borne. Malaria was a major source of morbidity and mortality across the tropical latitudes. It was also a fount of epidemiological puzzles, centring on the risk to unseasoned Europeans and migrant labour forces, and the often racist identification of 'native' populations and living conditions as a risk factor. The specific case of malaria is examined in detail in Chapter 8. By 1900, outbreaks of diseases such as bubonic plague in India and Brazil, sleeping sickness in central Africa and Chagas' disease in northern Brazil presented acute problems to those concerned with public and labour health, and international trade. The new tropical medicine seemed to promise a resolution to these problems.

In Europe, the contending work of Koch and Pasteur, igniting a controversy over the nature of the anthrax spore, stimulated a vibrant international network of medical scientists whose attentions soon began to shift to the research opportunities offered by tropical conditions. The growing prestige of medical microbiology, and the patronage of business and government interests enriched by the dynamic imperialism of the late nineteenth century, gave rise to institutions across the globe dedicated to tropical medicine. In 1899, the Liverpool and London Schools of Tropical Medicine were opened, while the next few years saw the foundation of institutes in tropical medicine in Hamburg and Paris in 1901 and Brussels in 1906. Chairs in Tropical Diseases and Medicine were endowed in Harvard and New Orleans, reflecting both the climatic diversity of the mainland United States and its expanded imperial role following the Spanish-American War in 1898. In Brazil, the Federal Seropathy Institute (later Oswaldo Cruz Institute), Manguinhos was founded in 1900, pioneering urban sanitation in Rio de Janeiro and spearheading scientific expeditions aimed at expanding the commercial potential of the Brazilian interior.

For many of its European practitioners, then, 'tropical medicine' was shorthand for novel clinical, sanitary and research responses to the demands of European adaptation to colonial conditions. Patrick Manson, the driving force behind the emergence of tropical medicine as a unified discipline in the British Empire, acknowledged as much when he noted that the term 'tropical diseases' was perhaps more a label of convenience than a description of a particular biological class of pathological organism. Consequently, the institutional development of tropical medicine, in the major ports and capitals of Europe as much as in colonial outposts, reflected the political as well as medical needs arising from European imperial activities. It is in this sense that tropical medicine has been described by Michael Worboys as occupying a 'residual category' among medical specialisms, 'synonymous with the additional requirements of imperial medical practice' (Worboys, 1993, p. 512).

Tropical medicine, then, was the predominant medical specialty addressing health concerns in areas of what we would now call the global South, characterized by a history of dependent relations with European and North American states and enterprises. This 'dependence' operated differently in Latin America, Africa, and South Asia, Southeast and East Asia. However, common themes emerge in the organization of labour, productivity and reproduction across a variety of colonies, trust territories, protectorates and independent states. As in the history of bacteriology and diagnostic medicine, the period 1880–1914 seems to have been significant across the global South. Public health initiatives, such as disease control programmes, capture some of the ambiguities and opportunities accompanying new relations of dependency in this period.

Exercise 5.3

The following edited excerpt is from a report on tropical medical problems in the Americas, as seen shortly after the outbreak of the First World War. The author's experience in Trinidad, an important source of cocoa and sugar for early twentieth century Britain, exemplifies the networks, forms of knowledge and approach to labour implicit in colonial tropical medicine. The author also comments on the habitat of the anopheles mosquito, the carrier of malaria, and on diseases such as leishmaniasis (kala-azar), endemic in India and associated with the South Asian labourers – known as 'coolies' in colonial terminology – who were brought in to work on plantations in the West Indies. Read the excerpt and then answer the questions that follow.

'There is much I might say about [Trinidad], our most important West Indian possession, for, in the stimulating company of Mr. URICH, the Government Entomologist, I ranged far and wide ... realising to the full the truth of these words –

"Where every prospect pleases
And only man is vile."

One is dealing with problems, however, not with prospects, so let me direct your attention to those which are, perhaps, the most interesting.

1 Why has kala-azar never been found in Trinidad, or, for that matter, in Jamaica? For many years a stream of East Indians, some of them from leishmaniasis areas, has been pouring into both these colonies. It is surely reasonable to suppose that amongst all these thousands of coolies some, when they left India, were in the incubation period of kala-azar, or were even in an early stage of the disease! Yet kala-azar has not been found ... is observation at fault, or is the insect-carrier absent? Personally, I am inclined to think the disease must be present and has not been recognised, but I saw nothing of it either in Trinidad or Jamaica, though, of course, my investigations were very limited.

2 There is a big scheme afoot for planting bamboo, as a source of paper pulp, on a large scale in Trinidad. How will this affect the malaria question there? Cut bamboos, unless severed at the nodes, leave ideal breeding places for anophelines. The hollow stem can, of course, be plugged with tar, but that would be a heavy task. Might something be done by having a cleared area round the plantation, and dotting trap-breeding pools here and there? This is at least worth thinking about.

3 Plague runs as an epizootic in rats. Can yellow fever exist as an epizootic in monkeys, and especially howler monkeys? I have already considered the possible

relationship of the indigenous monkeys of South America to obscure outbreaks of this disease, and Dr. LOW has replied to my hypothesis …On my way to the West Indies, I was told by a lady, Mrs. RANDOLPH RUST, who has been long resident in Trinidad, that the old negroes there say they can always tell when there is going to be an epidemic of yellow fever in the island owing to the fact that, prior to its appearance, the red howler monkeys are found dying and dead in the High Woods. In view of MANSON'S injunction to search for a reservoir of the virus amongst some of the lower animals, this negro statement struck me as curious and interesting, though naturally one did not place overmuch credence in it.'

(Balfour, 1915, pp. 86–7)

1 What does this excerpt tell us about the dissemination of expertise in tropical medicine?
2 What does the author identify as the most significant threat to health in the Americas?
3 What evidence is there for a preference of ecological and entomological [study of insects] approaches to disease control on the part of the author?
4 How is the non-European represented in the author's commentary? What, in your opinion, are the consequences of these representations for the discipline of tropical medicine?

Feedback

1 Balfour describes his meetings with a series of European commentators, scientists and clinicians in attempting to come to a formulation of the most significant problems in tropical health concerning Trinidad. He discusses a number of specific hypotheses, remarks on correspondence with other medical workers, and the significance of Patrick Manson's writing (see Chapter 8) in framing British tropical medical research agendas. Thus we can see evidence of the type of personal link, written correspondence and disciplinary architecture that was by this stage beginning to relate research in tropical medicine to problems in colonial governance.
2 The author is inclined to view migrant labour as a significant source of new infection. Despite his comments that leishmaniasis (kala-azar) had not emerged in either Jamaica or Trinidad, it is clear that he considers this to be a puzzle resolvable only by entomological enquiry, as the human reservoir was felt to be clearly present. His other hypotheses point to medical problems with roots in either local animal populations or the conditions of plantation agriculture. However, in all cases the agency of insects, whether explicit or implicit, is key.
3 Balfour exhibits a clear preference for ecological and entomological approaches to disease control: he seeks to identify insect vectors, and runs through a number of strategies for managing human–insect interactions, ranging from tarring cut stems to spatial management of breeding areas through tree-clearing and pool drainage. His emphasis is on interrupting or containing the non-human source of infection, whether insect or primate.
4 In this regard, the non-European is barely present in the universe of tropical medical intervention propounded by Balfour. Labour relations such as those involving coolies somehow streaming in from South Asia (the East Indies) are part of the backdrop against which disease control must be enacted, while the knowledge, observations and disease control strategies of long-resident Afro-Caribbean populations are easily discounted, even when corroborated or reported by a named European.

Efforts to control vector-borne diseases: Sleeping sickness

In the quarter century before the First World War, critics and proponents alike saluted the dynamism of imperial capitalism. The study and exploitation of new ecological niches, the development of tropical agriculture through networks of botanical gardens, and new urban environments and patterns of labour exploitation gave rise to unfamiliar issues in population management, food production and animal husbandry. The piecemeal and often contradictory approaches to managing the health implications of these systemic processes of change marked the emergent identity of the new tropical medicine in important ways.

The history of African trypanosomiasis (also known as sleeping sickness in humans and *nagana* in animals) is an exemplary case for an exploration of these issues. In the equatorial forest zones of West and Central Africa, the tsetse fly had long been noted as a barrier to the husbandry of large domestic animals such as horses, oxen and cattle. When it became clear in the early years of the twentieth century that some trypanosomes could affect both animals and humans, German and British scientists concerned with agricultural production and labour health in German Tanganyika and the sweep of British colonies from the Cape to the Horn of Africa began to investigate the least economically disruptive means of managing a catastrophic outbreak of epidemic sleeping sickness spreading across the Great Lakes region of Africa from 1896 – from Uganda into northern Tanganyika and southern Sudan (Ford, 1979; Bell, 1999).

Elsewhere, Europeans working in Africa, Asia and Latin America found themselves drawn into close relation with indigenous labour engaged in the harvesting of wild and plantation forest produce. In the last quarter of the nineteenth century and right up to the outbreak of the First World War, latex derived from wild rubber was a key commodity produced in European and North American industry. In Congo and across equatorial Africa, the exceptionally brutal labour conditions in rubber collection weakened human populations at the same time as exposing communities to the uncleared forest habitats of the tsetse fly. Local food production was undermined across the colonial equatorial forest zone, as labour exactions and colonial taxation accompanied rubber and palm produce booms. The toll on the health and nutrition of Africans enabled epidemic sleeping sickness to flourish across the Central and West Africa forest zone, and across the Great Lakes region of East Africa, engaging the scientific attentions of researchers from France, Belgium and Portugal (Lyons, 1992).

Over the two decades from 1901 (excluding 1914–1919) competing European scientific missions and control programmes went to work across Africa. British investigators isolated trypanosomal parasites in humans in the Gambia in 1901 and 1902 and, drawing on prior work on *nagana* by David Bruce, linked West and East African sleeping sickness, elucidating the role of the tsetse fly in its transmission. Robert Koch visited Tanganyika in 1905 to investigate the reservoir of the disease and potential chemotherapeutic treatments. An arsenical compound known as atoxyl emerged as the most suitable chemotherapeutic compound, and despite a relatively low success rate and high neurotoxicity, German and Portuguese clinicians promoted its extensive use.

The critical intervention of Belgian scientists in the role of King Leopold's brutal Congo Free State regime on the health of the Congolese contributed to the demise of the State and its annexation by the Belgian Government in 1908. Research on vector control and insect habitat, spearheaded by the British as a means of interrupting disease transmission (eliminating the insect from the transmission cycle), was also carried out by Portuguese missions to Angola and the plantation island of Principe. Here, and in British East Africa and northern Nigeria, the vector control approach to combating infectious tropical disease was worked out to its fullest extent (Tilley, 2004). This culminated in proposals to cull game and animal reservoirs, inviting resistance from European settler farmers and African pastoralists alike.

Post-1910 French missions to equatorial Africa took a different approach to disease control. Eugène Jamot evolved a method of systematic case detection, population screening and the mass administration of arsenicals (eliminating the parasite from the host), with military backing, which he deployed in response to the 1916 Brazzaville epidemic of sleeping sickness. Later, he also deployed it in endemic sleeping sickness in Cameroon, which had largely been entrusted to French control after the defeat of the German Empire in the First World War. The contrast between ecological-entomological and population-screening approaches to disease control was to be a prominent feature of tropical medicine throughout the colonial period, and continues to inform contemporary public health approaches to epidemic disease.

Missionary medicine

Throughout the European colonial encounter with the territories of the tropical latitudes, the impact of Christian missionary medical work on public health was central to overall health care provision. The impact of medical research carried out by missionaries was largely limited to the arena of leprosy control. However, in the areas of maternal and child health, and rural health, the missionary contribution was crucial in defining the character and range of colonial medical practice, and the scope of tropical public health planning. The medical missionary was also a central character in the dramatization of tropical medicine – in the hands of the missionary, the labours involved in addressing the physical and spiritual needs of the impoverished and ignorant native of the tropics became charged with images of the redemptive and noble nature of the work.

The vision of the missionary represented a wide range of apparently altruistic concerns with welfare and public health in the tropical latitudes. Contemporary missionary literature suggests that medical work was seen as a powerful exemplar of Christ's love. As an evangelical tool, medical mission seems to have been of dubious effect overall, whatever its sporadic local successes. However, as a material contributor to the extension of rural public health, and as a source of information on rural conditions, this work was highly significant in the overall meagre profile of colonial concern for rural health outside the plantation.

The critical contribution of the medical missionary was the focus on conditions of poverty, and the local and predominantly rural nature of missionary work. The lifestyle and work of the medical missionary was based on a close and ongoing association with agrarian communities, which brought hospital and outpatient medicine to many otherwise neglected areas of Africa, China and India, and engaged in the initial recruitment and training of local medical dressers, nurses and technicians (see, for example, Kumwenda, 2006).

The visibility of Western biomedicine, manifested on a human scale by missionaries, increased greatly in the period from 1919 to 1939. The suspicions prompted by militaristic and coercive campaigns of early tropical medicine were not entirely supplanted by missionary and indigenous medical workers (Hunt, 1999). However, the missionary emphasis on resolving the complications of poverty (if not necessarily challenging its roots), together with their substantial field experience, provided a critical complement to the often less than satisfactory public health interventions of colonial states.

Exercise 5.4

This painting below represents the medical work of the missionary in rural Africa in the heyday of Protestant medical mission. Christian mission worked hard at distinguishing itself from other spiritual traditions of healing active in Africa and Asia. It was not unusual for a visiting medical worker to set up stall close to a village meeting area, and many depictions of missionary and public health work in Africa include a prominent tree in proximity to the clearing where the health workers operate. Look closely at the drama presented in the painting and then answer the questions that follow.

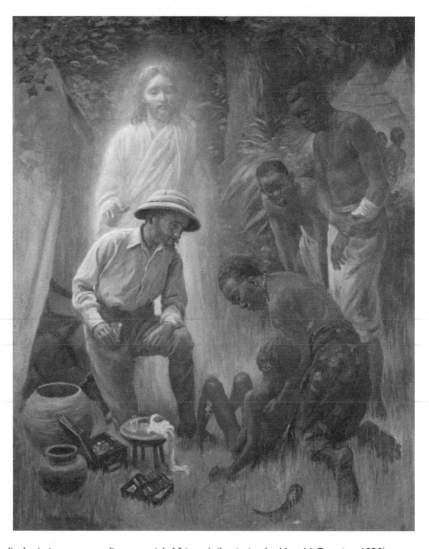

Figure 5.2 A medical missionary attending to a sick African (oil painting by Harold Copping, 1930)
Credit: Wellcome Library, London

1 From what does the doctor's power and status derive?
2 How are the major threats to health represented in the painting?
3 What do you think the spiritual power of the missionary added to medical work?
4 Who is the painting for?

Feedback

1 A number of elements in the painting's depiction of the therapeutic setting stand out as evidence of the doctor figure's power and status. The benign – and invisible – presence of Christ the Healer at his shoulder is the clearest indication of blessings on the missionary's work, but the wonder we see in the eyes of the watching men relates to the visible healing process, set in motion with a remedy selected, prepared and administered from boxes of surgical tools, bandages and pharmaceuticals. Together with these materials, the doctor's clothing, headgear, stool and sheltered seat create the sense of a distinct therapeutic space.

2 The painting depicts a number of threats to health. The amazement of the family figures accompanying the patient can be taken to represent curiosity and gratitude for missionary work, at the same time as depicting the threat of ignorance to the health of the young African. The line of sight of the missionary is perhaps deliberately ambiguous: while observing clinical signs and patient response, does he see what may be the menacing figure of a snake that approaches the mother's unusually large and uncovered foot? White marks on the skin of the child and the mother figure may depict the treatment for skin ailments that formed a significant proportion of cases treated by missionary medical workers. We might also read the proximity of two thatched local houses in the background gloom as evidence of conditions of over-crowding held responsible for much rural ill health.

3 Spirituality and serenity may lie behind the missionary's power to work wonders and to calm the apprehension and suspicion of the family figures. Is the conversing pair in the background discussing the status and progress of the doctor's works? Their expectant stance may suggest an intense desire for powerful new therapies – this was certainly the sense derived by missionaries from experiences such as that depicted in the picture.

4 This painting is for a range of audiences. Missionaries were of vital importance in producing propaganda and rhetoric linking Western 'publics' to the pursuit of better public health in Asia and Africa. This painting depicts all the skills and the spiritual glories and consolations of medical missionary work to an avid donor audience as engaged by colonial as by religious dramas. Also, the role of missionary propaganda in recruiting the next generation of spiritual adventurers for the souls of Africa and Asia cannot be overlooked.

The rise of philanthropy

The technical and advisory work promulgated through the 1910s and 1920s in the treatment of hookworm in the southern USA, Latin America and the Philippines by the Rockefeller Foundation has been strongly associated with the global projection of American power (Cueto, 1994); indeed, its philanthropic profile is very different to that of the diverse universe of missionary groups that sought to preach and enact a Christian model of healing. Concerned in the United States with the vitality of southern labour, the

Rockefeller Foundation pioneered a programme of public health interventions designed to be agnostic as to social structure and systemic inequality, while at the same time improving population health through well organized and technically feasible health interventions.

The success of the hookworm programme before the First World War in the United States prompted Rockefeller strategists to promote hookworm research and treatment across Latin America, providing governments with much-needed public health funding and the promise of capacity-building in training and maintaining indigenous expertise. This rarely came to pass, and Rockefeller programmes were accused of restructuring public health across Latin America, and diluting state sovereignty over health services across the region. The technocratic approach they pioneered was to prove increasingly influential later in the twentieth century, as will be demonstrated in Chapter 11.

Neither missionary nor philanthropic approaches to tropical health mounted a substantial challenge to the roots of tropical health inequalities. Nor did tropical medicine, for all its technical innovation, entirely overcome prior associations between tropical bodies and locales, and dangerous and unpredictable disease terrain. The persistence of expensive segregatory approaches to urban sanitation and disease control demonstrate that germ theory did not completely supplant spatial and miasmatic ideas of population management and disease control. 'Race' continued to be a powerful influence on European thinking about disease in indigenous populations. From nineteenth-century ideas of the dying race, generated through ideas of racial immunity seemingly supported by relatively high morbidity and mortality rates among Europeans from malaria, to ideas of detribalization among urban dwellers ostensibly torn from the social and political supports of their own communities, notions of race were key to understanding European colonial medicine.

The intersection of race and public health received its most potent formulation in the relation between skin, sexuality and urban population health. The conceptual and diagnostic confusion surrounding leprosy, yaws and syphilis emerges again and again through the first half of the twentieth century, always enveloped in distressed considerations of racial intimacy, difference and danger (Vaughan, 1992). Whatever the promises of tropical medicine, the world in which its practitioners studied, researched and operated continued to be shaped by the uneasy and compromising conditions of imperial rule, philanthropic endeavour and ecological exploitation.

Exercise 5.5

Read the following excerpt from *An African Survey* (1938) on health in Africa and then answer the questions that follow.

'Public attention and public sympathy, from the days of Livingstone [generally held to be the first British medical missionary in Africa, arriving in South Africa in 1841] onwards, have been concentrated upon the grave diseases such as leprosy, sleeping sickness, and malaria, from which in Africa there is widespread suffering, and alleviation of these sufferings has been the prime object of medical aid and of public philanthropy. The realisation of another approach is rapidly gaining ground ...

Medical science must be in Africa increasingly concerned with the relations between nutrition and health, and with advising on the medical aspect of social policies bearing on the question of subsistence. In the second place, the fact that there is one widely prevalent factor which, by reducing the power of resistance, favours the widespread existence of disease, suggests the conclusion that the methods applied by health services must be largely those of mass attack. The preventive treatment applied to certain of the African diseases, to be effective, must partake to some extent of the character of an operation, scientifically planned and humanely conducted, but military in its spirit of offensive and the thoroughness with which it establishes itself in the area it has occupied. There is a third point; the narrowness of the financial resources available, which in Europe would appear almost derisory in view of the scope of the operations to be undertaken, requires that, under a scientific leadership, there should be a large body of assistants, who must as far as possible be Africans, and who must have as complete a system of training as circumstances will permit. The scope of activity of the health services in Africa is not, therefore, confined to the application of the lessons which modern science conveys of the causes of disease by the method of relieving it. There is added to that the task of organising to the best purpose of the narrow resources which the state can place at their disposal, the education of Africans to take part in health activities, and the cooperation with the other social services whose work lies in the betterment of African conditions of life.'

(Lord Hailey, 1938, pp. 1114–15)

1   How does the author account for the constrained focus of tropical medicine to date, and how does he propose to address this?
2   The author is optimistic about the prospects for African health. Why?
3   What is the most important cause of ill-health, as described in the extract? Do the author's proposals appear likely to address this cause? Explain your answer.

Feedback

1   The author demonstrates that (British) public opinion had long focused on the grave diseases identified by missionaries such as Livingstone and other proponents of tropical medicine and, more specifically, on the suffering they caused. His proposals include mass prevention campaigns, drawing on the range of social services provided in the colonies, and training an extensive cohort of African medical workers. Note that the scale of this enterprise is shown to be cost-effective, presumably relying on the great disparity between European and African wages in British colonies. Likewise, the role of scientific (and presumably European) supervision is important in maintaining what is proposed as the military character of the venture.
2   The excerpt is suffused with the sense that key health problems have now been identified, and that an ideal cost-effective and technically feasible strategy for overcoming these problems is clearly available. While the resources of the state are patently 'narrow', the differentiation of services concerned with 'the betterment of African conditions of life' would seem to the author adequate to the scale of the educational, social and medical enterprise to be undertaken.
3   However, apart from identifying the relations between nutrition and health at the heart of the conundrum for medical science in Africa, the author proposes little of direct relevance to addressing nutritional deficit. The thoroughness of preventive interventions, and the degree to which they take root in an area, is hoped to be sufficient to combat the 'widespread existence of disease', without expressly combating the factor which '[reduces] the power of resistance'. While this excerpt points to a readjustment of colonial attitudes to population health, and shows evidence of a

feedback from forty years of field experience in tropical medicine into policy, it is not as fully integrated a vision of public health as the author supposes.

Summary

At the outbreak of the Second World War, after a long period of economic depression, systematic public health interventions were beyond the capacity of most colonial states. While social medicine (discussed in more detail in Chapter 10) had made substantial inroads in South Africa, health coverage in much of Africa and India was still only sporadic, and such public health visions as there were proved no more than aspirational. Great strides had been made in microbiology, in techniques of disease management and control, and increasingly in chemotherapy. But the draconian nature of many of the measures employed in managing epidemics and populations highlighted the grave inequalities that persisted under the extractive nature of colonial capitalism.

The roots of tropical medicine were inspired by the dreams and needs of Europeans, as much as in the scientific and technical advances accompanying the rise of imperialism. Colonial logics, missionary as much as capitalist, continued to shape the specialism of tropical medicine that would only begin to break down as colonial empires began to unravel after the Second World War. This very different world will be examined in Chapter 11. But, as we will see in the next chapter, disease control posed dilemmas in the West just as it did in the global South.

References and further reading

Balfour A (1915) Tropical problems in the New World, *Transactions of the Royal Society of Tropical Medicine and Hygiene*, 8(3): 75–108.

Bell H (1999) *Frontiers of Medicine in the Anglo-Egyptian Sudan, 1899–1940*. Oxford Historical Monographs. Oxford: Clarendon Press.

Chandavarkar R (1992) Plague panic and epidemic politics in India 1896–1914, in Ranger T and Slack P (eds) *Epidemics and Ideas: Essays on the Historical Perception of Pestilence* (pp. 199–236). Cambridge: Cambridge University Press.

Cueto M (1994) *Missionaries of Science: The Rockefeller Foundation and Latin America*. Bloomington, IN: Indiana University Press.

Curtin P (1989) *Death by Migration: Europe's Encounter with the Tropical World in the Nineteenth Century*. Cambridge: Cambridge University Press.

Dobson M (1980) 'Marsh fever' – the geography of malaria in England, *Journal of Historical Geography*, 6(4): 357–89.

Drayton R (2000) *Nature's Government: Science, Imperial Britain, and the Improvement of the World*. New Haven, CT: Yale University Press.

Felkin RW (1889) *On the Geographical Distribution of Some Tropical Diseases, and Their Relation to Physical Phenomena*. Edinburgh: Young J. Pentland.

Ford J (1979) Ideas which have influenced attempts to solve the problems of African trypanosomiasis, *Social Science and Medicine, Part B: Medical Anthropology*, 13(4): 269–75.

Hailey, Lord (1938) *An African Survey: A Study of the Problems Arising in Africa South of the Sahara*. London: Oxford University Press.

Hardiman D (2006) Introduction, in Hardiman D (ed) *Healing Bodies, Saving Souls: Medical Missions in Asia and Africa* (pp. 5–57). Amsterdam: Rodopi.

Harrison M (2005) Science and the British empire, *Isis*, 96: 56–63.

Hunt N (1999) *A Colonial Lexicon of Birth Ritual, Medicalization, and Mobility in the Congo*. Durham, NC: Duke University Press.

Kumwenda L (2006) African medical personnel of the Universities' Mission to Central Africa in Northern Rhodesia, in Hardiman D (ed) *Healing Bodies, Saving Souls: Medical Missions in Asia and Africa* (pp. 193–226). Amsterdam: Rodopi.

Lyons M (1992) *The Colonial Disease: A Social History of Sleeping Sickness in Northern Zaire, 1900–40*. Cambridge: Cambridge University Press.

Stepan N (2006) *Picturing Tropical Nature*. London: Reaktion Books.

Tilley H (2004) Ecologies of complexity: Tropical environments, African trypanosomiasis, and the science of disease control in British Colonial Africa, 1900–1940, *Osiris*, 19 (2nd Ser.): 21–38.

Vaughan M (1992) Syphilis in colonial east and central Africa: The social construction of an epidemic, in Ranger T and Slack P (eds) *Epidemics and Ideas: Essays on the Historical Perception of Pestilence* (pp. 269–302). Cambridge: Cambridge University Press.

Worboys M (1993) Tropical diseases, in Bynum WF and Porter R (eds) *Companion Encyclopaedia of the History of Medicine* (pp. 512–36). London: Routledge.

SECTION 2

Case studies

Case study: Sexual health

Virginia Berridge

6

Overview

As we have shown in previous chapters, the history of disease control highlights many key issues in the development of public health in the tropics and in the West. A particularly problematic set of conditions relate to sexual health (the modern term), which have posed dilemmas for societies since ancient times. The phrase 'venereal disease' was coined in the 1520s but sexually transmitted diseases (STDs) can be traced back to biblical times. It is likely that gonorrhoea existed in Europe and the Middle East before the fifteenth century, when syphilitic infections probably first arrived from the New World. In recent times, the issue of HIV/AIDS has brought sexual health onto policy agendas in high, middle and low income countries.

Learning objectives

After working through this chapter, you will be able to:

- describe how historical and cultural contexts have shaped responses to STDs
- use primary source material to identify and explain some of the factors involved in shaping responses to STDs
- distinguish between different policy responses to STDs and evaluate the reasons why these were introduced

Key terms

Gonorrhoea Caused by a bacterium, *Neisseria gonorrheae*, with an incubation period of between two and ten days. Infection is often unaccompanied by symptoms, but most common evidence is local genital discharge. Chronic infection can cause more long-term complications such as chronic pelvic pain (pelvic inflammatory disease) and sub-fertility.

Sexually transmitted disease (STD) A recent term used to cover what used to be called venereal disease.

Introduction

In the last three decades, the arrival and spread of HIV/AIDS has drawn attention to the impact of sexually transmitted diseases on society and the dilemmas that their control can bring. Sexually transmitted diseases (STDs) have affected societies since the earliest times. Control of STDs has embodied dilemmas about the competing demands of individual liberty versus the common good of society. They have been seen as threats to the basis of society, expressing fears about class, race, sexuality and the family. As we will see, different societies have responded in different ways to the threat of STDs. When HIV/AIDS came on the agenda, the ways in which STDs had been responded to helped to inform initial responses to HIV/AIDS in some countries. In this chapter, we will investigate how and why STDs have been responded to.

Exercise 6.1

A range of options for the control of STDs is provided below. Examine these and then think about the current way in which STDs are controlled in the country in which you live. Give reasons why you think STDs are responded to in this way.

Confidential medical treatment   Partner notification   Compulsory testing

◄───►

Feedback

Depending on where you live, you will have highlighted different forms of response. These can even vary within countries if there is a federal system of government. For example, some states in the United States have premarital tests for STDs while others do not. At the time of writing Mississippi, Colorado and the District of Columbia still had this requirement on their statute books. Responses have also changed over time. In Britain in the nineteenth century there was a punitive policy focused on controlling prostitutes. Later, this changed to a more liberal policy. Thus responses cannot be placed within fixed time categories; these have changed with place and time.

Your reasons for the positioning of STDs may include factors such as:

• the perceived level of spread within society;
• the association with prostitution or with women's or family health;
• the dangers posed to society;
• vested interests such as the medical profession.

We will return to consider these factors at the end of the chapter.

Early history

Syphilis was the first sexually transmitted disease to be heard of in European countries at the end of the fifteenth century. An invasion of Naples by Charles VIII of France led to an outbreak among troops and camp followers. Mercenaries then spread the disease throughout Europe, where it became endemic. Even in these early times, an enduring feature of the response emerged: this was the need to blame others for the spread of the disease. So the Italians called it 'the French disease' or 'Morbus Gallicus', while the

French called it the 'Italian disease'. Historians have debated whether syphilis was introduced to Europe by the explorer Christopher Columbus and his followers on their return from the discovery of America and the 'New World'. This was part of what has been called the 'Columbian exchange' of diseases between the Old World in Europe and the New in the Americas (Crosby, 1972). There has also been discussion of whether syphilis changed its nature. The organism of syphilis is like that for yaws, a tropical disease, and there has been speculation that it acquired its present nature when man migrated to cooler areas.

Exercise 6.2

Examine the drawing below of a man with syphilis by the German artist Albrecht Dürer in the late fifteenth century. What message is the artist trying to convey about people who have the disease?

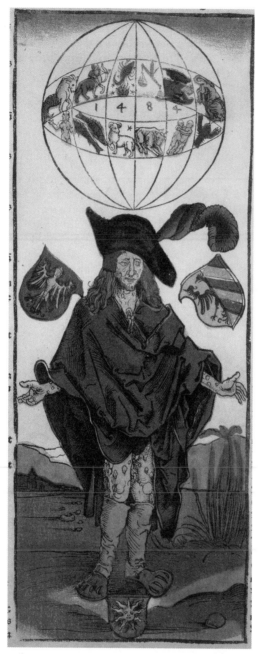

Figure 6.1 Detail of a syphilitic person from Broadsheet: Syphilitic; woodcut ascribed to Albrecht Dürer Woodcut and text by Albrecht Dürer (1496)

Credit: Wellcome Library, London

Feedback

The drawing shows the unpleasant physical manifestations of the disease. The man has sores on his legs. But he is also portrayed in a particular way, with fashionable clothing, a feather in his hat. He is a 'man about town' who is suffering for his sexual habits. Dürer, who was German, also portrays him as a Frenchman, an example of the way in which the disease was blamed on what historians call 'the other', people different from ourselves. The drawing is headed by signs of the zodiac, which stress the sign of the scorpion, said to rule the genitalia. This illustrates the importance given to astrological influences in the understanding of disease at this time.

Treatment for diseases like syphilis was limited and mercury was widely used, a risky undertaking, which led to ulcerated jaws and mouths and loosened teeth. In London, there were 'mercury wards' from the sixteenth century in two hospitals, St. Thomas' and St. Bartholomew's. Later, specialist hospitals developed. These were called 'Lock' hospitals, the name coming from 'loques', the bandages or lint worn over the syphilitic sores.

Dilemmas of regulation

How to control what were called 'venereal diseases' became an issue for societies in particular in the nineteenth century. Concern about the possible weakening of the army and military effort because of the impact of venereal diseases grew, a concern given added urgency by the development of tropical empires where troops were regularly deployed at a distance from their home country. The fear was that they might import the disease on their return or it might weaken the imperial mission. This is a theme of note within public health and medicine: initiatives in research, innovations in medicine, and also policy responses to health issues have often had their origin in a desire to protect the health of fighting men. Indeed, venereal disease was widespread in the ranks of the British army in Victorian times: 31 per cent of the army in Bengal was infected in the late 1820s. There was also concern that troops returning from the Empire could spread the disease at home.

Concern about venereal disease was fuelled by additional fear about the widespread nature of prostitution in Victorian society. There was an obsession with this 'social evil' in the 1850s and 1860s. The standard image of the sex trade is that of middle-class men debauching working-class women, but there was also a widespread working-class trade. Historians have shown that being a prostitute was not a set occupation for some working-class women but rather part of a range of sexual activities that were fluid and changed over time (Walkowitz, 1980).

Different countries took different stances in the nineteenth century on what was the most appropriate form of regulation. In Britain, it was not illegal to sell sexual services and there were no regulatory systems as in parts of Europe and North America. Some nations took the line that society was best served by the provision of healthy prostitutes: prostitutes were licensed in France.

But regulation could also be intensely controversial. The Contagious Diseases Acts in Britain in the second half of the nineteenth century are an illustration of this. These Acts, passed in 1864, 1866 and 1869, were inspired by more stringent European systems and aimed at the eradication of venereal disease in the army. They instituted strict regulation, medical examination and policing of prostitutes in military areas, but not the men with whom they had relations. The women could be forcibly treated and confined until they were free of disease.

Exercise 6.3

Read the quotation below from an official enquiry into these Acts which reported in 1871, and then answer the questions that follow.

'...there is no comparison to be made between prostitutes and the men who consort with them. With the one sex the offence is committed as a matter of gain; with the other it is an irregular indulgence of a natural impulse.'

(Royal Commission on the Contagious Diseases Acts, 1871)

1 What message is this statement conveying?
2 What is your view of this quotation? Do you think it is a fair assessment of the situation?

Feedback

The official report exonerates men from any blame and sees their sexual activity as natural, a brief fall from grace. Women, on the other hand, are seen as blameworthy. Their activity is driven by economics, not impulse; they are the guilty parties in the transaction. This attitude formed the basis of what became known as the 'double standard' of morality in the nineteenth century: it made a clear differentiation between the sexes.

In assessing such attitudes it is easy to be condemnatory in turn. However, comments such as these must also be assessed in the context of the time. We discuss below some of the historical interpretations of these Acts.

Historians' interpretations of regulation

A campaign against the Contagious Diseases Acts was led by the activist Josephine Butler and her organization, the Ladies' National Association. Their imagery, which stressed the 'instrumental rape' of poor women through forcible examination, was effective, and the Acts were repealed in 1886. Historians have seen the significance of the Acts in different ways: this case study illustrates the way in which interpretation of events in history can vary.

Historians writing from a feminist perspective have seen the campaign against them as part of the history of women's social and political emancipation (Walkowitz and Walkowitz, 1974). But the Acts were also part of a new set of relationships between medicine and the state. The historian Frank Mort argues that their significance was in helping to produce an alliance between the medical profession and the state. He writes: '... the acts implicated the state and medical expertise in a much more precise and extensive discourse on sexuality ... part of the intensified scrutiny of female behaviour and the sexual habits of the urban poor' (Mort, 2000, p. 57). This view stresses the negative aspects of regulation. But the Australian historian F.B. Smith has taken a different view. He points out that repressive regulation could have positive health benefits. The Acts could have contributed to the fall in cases of neonatal ophthalmia (an eye infection contracted by newborns from the mother, most often caused by STDs) between 1871 and 1891, from 951 per million to 809 per million, the fastest fall in the century (Smith, 1990). Smith criticized the opponents of the Acts for what he called 'parasitic sanctified narcissism'. Such divergence in historical assessment also illustrates some of the dilemmas of regulation. Punitive and inequitable regulation could also, as in this case, have had some positive health benefits. Societies have to decide what the trade-off in these cases will be.

Population fears and birth control

Towards the end of the nineteenth century, a new fear – about the population and its quality – came on to the agenda (as we show in Chapter 10). The birth rate began to decline from the 1870s onwards, initially among the middle class. There were a variety of reasons for this. Birth control and the reduction in the size of families contributed to the maintenance of standards of living, which could be dragged down by having to support large numbers of children. There were new attitudes towards women, who were beginning to emerge from the home and to play a role in public life, and also a new view of children. Parents had previously expected that quite large numbers of their children would die at a young age. There was a fatalistic attitude and also less emotional involvement with children and 'childhood' as a stage of life. But this also began to change. As children became fewer in number, they became more precious to their parents.

Birth control, helping to bring this state of affairs about, was a controversial matter. Those who wrote birth control literature were liable to prosecution. Free thinkers and secularists were prominent in promoting limitation of births and the Malthusian League, which promoted the views of the political economist Thomas Malthus, was also active in this field. One famous trial was of the reformers Charles Bradlaugh and Annie Besant in 1877 for publishing *The Fruits of Philosophy*, a pamphlet by American physician John Knowlton that provided advice on birth control.

Behind the concern about population decline and birth control was a fear about what was called the differential birth rate – that the middle class would limit their births while the working class would not. At the turn of the century, there were fears about what was then called the 'residuum', a section of society that might now be termed the 'underclass'. There was concern that this unhealthy section of society, equated with the lower classes, would come to predominate in the nation through extensive reproduction, while the more refined middle class would shrink because of the adoption of birth control.

It used to be assumed that the change in the birth rate was part of different relationships within the family, and the rise of what has been called 'companionate marriage'. Women were taking charge of birth control and were no longer willing to put up with endless pregnancies and the health problems that resulted. But the evidence seemed to show that most women were ignorant of birth control. Oral history interviews with working-class men and women have thrown light on how and why birth control was used. They have shown that relationships within marriage were more complex and there was negotiation over sexual matters. Women's apparent ignorance could be assumed for cultural reasons to avoid the appearance of sexual knowledge. It mattered for a wife to show ignorance because to know about such matters could be seen as sleazy (Fisher, 2006). Historians have also drawn attention to the use of coitus interruptus (sexual intercourse deliberately interrupted by withdrawal of the penis from the vagina prior to ejaculation) as a major means of birth control (Szreter, 1995). These investigations have underlined that the adoption of birth control was a complex matter and that the influence of birth control reformers and their information was only a part of a fundamental shift in personal relationships.

Medical progress

The turn of the century was also marked by significant scientific and medical progress; part of the 'laboratory revolution' (discussed in Chapter 3) that saw the understanding of disease transformed in many areas. For the first time, the organisms causing venereal diseases were identified and it became possible to begin to develop more effective treatments and also preventive measures. These positive steps also brought fresh dilemmas, which highlighted the continuing tensions inherent in responses to STDs.

In 1879, Albert Neisser, a German, discovered the causative organism of gonorrohoea, *Neisseria gonorrhoeae*. In 1905, the causative organism of syphilis, *Treponema pallidum*, was identified by Fritz Shaudinn and Erich Hoffmann and in 1906, August Wassermann, Albert Neisser, Carl Bruck and other German scientists developed a serological test for the organism. In 1909, Paul Ehrlich and his Japanese coworker Sahachiro Hata synthesized an arsenical compound that they called Salvarsan and which opened up the possibility of 'cure' for the first time. Ehrlich's compound was the 606th arsenical he had synthesized. It symbolized a new world of biomedicine in which 'magic bullets' would target and eliminate disease. This drug was the main treatment for STDs until the advent of penicillin in the 1940s. Other advances also took place. Work by Metchnikoff and Roux proved that inoculation with the syphilitic virus could be rendered inactive by applying calomel in ointment within a few hours of infection. This tactic was tried in Europe, in France and Germany in particular, in the early years of the twentieth century. It opened up a new dilemma in the response to STDs, that of potentially 'condoning' immorality by offering treatment and prevention either before or after the sexual act.

Exercise 6.4

Examine the painting below, a watercolour representing syphilis by Richard Cooper, part of a series painted for Sir Henry Wellcome, the pharmaceutical manufacturer who also had a strong interest in history and anthropology. After you have examined it, answer the questions that follow.

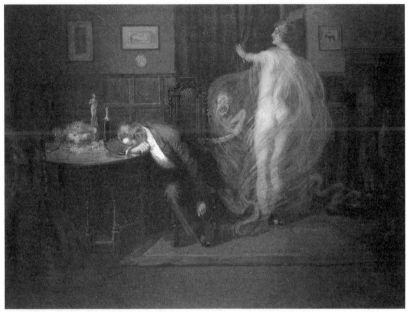

Figure 6.2 'Syphilis', 1910, by Richard Cooper

Credit: Wellcome Library, London

1 What does the painting convey about the impact of syphilis?
2 What do you think about the portrayal of the woman and of the man?
3 The image was painted in 1910. Can you think why this timing may be significant?

Feedback

1 Although medical advance was being made and the nature of the organism and infection was understood at the time this painting was completed, the picture does not convey optimism but rather despair. The man sitting at the table may have just had the news that he is infected with syphilis: is it clear that he is devastated. This reminds us that medical advance in the laboratory is not immediately translated into public understanding or use of treatment. At this stage the diagnosis was still overwhelmingly negative and a potential death sentence.

2 The woman is presented as the seductress; she is to blame. In fact, the imagery of her in the nude is semi-pornographic by the standards of the time. This reminds us that condemnation and salacious enjoyment of sexual matters are often two sides of the same coin. The small 'hobgoblin' in the painting may represent the hidden disease

that she is harbouring, or the loss of beauty and the horror that the ravages of syphilis will bring to both of them. The man, on the other hand, is clearly from an upper- or middle-class background. His room is well furnished and he is wearing evening dress. His social status underlines the contemporary fear that 'respectable society' would be undermined by the spread of STDs.

3 The date of 1910 is significant because the early twentieth century was the time when fears about the quality of the population and the decline of the middle class were at their height. The representations in the painting underline these fears and help to heighten them.

The impacts of war and of medicine on regulation

The First World War, and the attention focused on the impact of STDs on civilian and military health, brought the dilemmas of scientific advance to a head. Many countries began to introduce what became seen as the public health approach of education: early diagnosis, notification, contact tracing and the provision of treatment. In Britain, a Royal Commission to enquire into the subject had been appointed before the war, but war added urgency to the issue of venereal disease. In 1916, an order from the Army Council required troops to attend for disinfection within twenty-four hours of sexual infection. But it was argued that such a system of prophylaxis was not intended to afford 'opportunities for unrestrained vice'. The pretence was that ablution was not for prevention but for treatment. The issue of 'condoning vice' or not was one that divided organizations working in this field. The issue was summed up as follows: should disinfection occur at 10.45 pm, before the act had taken place, or at 11.15 pm, afterwards? In Britain, the end result at the national level was confirmation of a medicalized and confidential response to STDs. A network of treatment centres was set up to which patients could refer themselves. These were free and mainly funded by government working through the local authorities. This was a harbinger of a new attitude towards the provision of a state medical service that would ultimately result in the National Health Service (NHS).

Exercise 6.5

The following is an extract from the Final Report of the Royal Commission on Venereal Diseases (1917). Read through the extract and then answer the questions that follow.

'Our task is now ended. We have endeavoured to make clear the grave and far reaching effects of venereal disease upon the individual and the race. The evidence that we have taken proves conclusively that these effects cannot be too seriously regarded, and that they result in a heavy loss, not only of actual but of potential population, of productive power and of expenditure actually entailed ...

The medical evidence establishes the fact that, by early and efficient treatment, these diseases could be brought under control and reduced within narrow limits ... Recent discoveries have armed the medical profession with means of combating venereal disease which were unknown in the past. The object must be to bring these means to bear upon every infected person at the earliest possible moment.

We are convinced that this object can be accomplished only by the action of Government directed to the solution of a great national problem. We have recom-

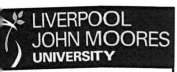

LIVERPOOL JOHN MOORES UNIVERSITY

).. *364 119* ...

Self Collection of holds

st 6 digits of barcode no.
ocated on the bottom of
your University card

ease issue the item
at the self service
machine before you
leave this area.

u.ac.uk   **LIBRARY SERVICES**

no drastic remedies, and except in certain special cases we have not advo-
ompulsion in any form. The measures which we propose contemplate
d facilities for bacteriological diagnosis combined with the provision of
e and skilled free treatment, the cost of which, we consider, should fall
n the national exchequer …

erms of our reference precluded consideration of the moral aspects of the
s with which we have dealt. We are, however, deeply sensible of the need
ortance of the appeals to conscience and honour which are made by the
bodies and by associations formed for this purpose. We believe that these
will gain force if the terrible effects of venereal disease upon innocent chil-
d other persons who have no vicious tendencies are more fully realised.
dence tends to show that the communication of disease is frequently due
gence in intoxicants, and there is no doubt that the growth of temperance
the population would help to bring about an amelioration of the very seri-
ditions which our enquiry has revealed. We are also conscious of the fact
ercrowded and insanitary dwellings indirectly contribute to the spread of
…

re, therefore, convinced that it will not suffice to establish treatment centres
s where soldiers and sailors are congregated, and that these will be needed
of the larger and in some of the smaller towns. We realise the claims of
economy at the present moment; but, for reason we have given, we believe that all
necessary expenditure will be recouped by the results which can be obtained.

Lastly, we wish to pay stress upon the need of the future. The diminution of the
best manhood of the nation, due to the losses of the war, must tell heavily upon the
birth rate – already declining – and upon the numbers of efficient workers … Now
and in the years to come the question of public health must be a matter of para-
mount national importance, and no short sighted parsimony should be permitted
to stand in the way of all means that science can suggest and organisation can supply
for guarding the present and future generations upon which the restoration of
national prosperity must depend.'

(Report of the Royal Commission on Venereal Disease, P.P. 1916, Cd. 8189 XVI,
Plate VIII and pp. 65–6)

1 Why are main concerns of the signatories to this report about venereal disease?
2 What additional issues have been involved in the spread of venereal disease?
3 What does the report see as the solution to the problem?

Feedback

1 The main concerns include the effects upon the individual but also of the population
as a whole. The report is concerned that venereal disease will undermine the productive capacity of the nation. Economic argument – mentions of economic efficiency –
figures largely. The report is also concerned about the quality of the population and
the effect of venereal disease on the birth rate, which is already in decline. There is
concern about the impact on soldiers and sailors but the concern goes wider than
that, to the whole population. There is particular anxiety about the impact on 'innocent victims' such as children, who have been infected involuntarily, through no fault
of their own. This focus on 'innocent victims' is a common theme in public health, in
sexual health especially, and came to the fore again in the response to HIV/AIDS.

2 Additional factors have included intemperance and also the state of housing and living conditions. In this way, the report is ascribing both individual failings and more general social conditions as being implicated in the spread of venereal disease.

3 The report places emphasis on science and medicine and also on the role of the state in providing a national network of treatment centres. It represents the new faith in government action in health at this period and also the growing reliance on what medicine and science could provide.

National differences in response

Different nations adopted different strategies to control the diseases. Britain's approach was not universally replicated. In France and Germany, there was regulation tempered by eventual reform (Sauerteig, 2001). Scandinavian countries such as Sweden aimed to regulate the entire population and had rigorous measures for the tracing of infected persons. In the United States, a major campaign was instituted during the 1930s to enforce diagnosis and treatment of venereal diseases. There, the issue had a racial dimension and syphilis in particular was seen as an African-American problem. Pre-marital blood tests for all racial groups were put in place in the 1930s and were used to prevent marriage of those who were infected (Brandt, 1985). So, scientific advance in this area did not result in a universal policy model for STDs. The policies that were put in place depended on factors other than science. These included whether political cultures were liberal or authoritarian; relationships with the military system; and social politics and the influence of activist organizations. As in other areas, these variables lay behind the impact of scientific understanding.

Colonial models

Historians have noted that the economics and politics of colonialism also influenced the spread of STDs and the ways in which policy responses developed (Lewis and Bamber, 1997). Economic growth and urbanization created the preconditions for the use of sexual labour in prostitution. Different European countries adopted different regulatory models but so, too, did colonial countries. The nineteenth-century system of compulsory treatment of prostitutes was introduced by colonial states. The Contagious Diseases Acts operated in some countries in distinctive imperial versions. In the colonies such regulation was aimed at protecting the military and also the resident colonists rather than the indigenous population. There were fears about 'African sexuality' and contacts with 'other races'. There was concern about soldiers returning home and transmitting infection. Sometimes models that operated in the colonies were at variance with the regulation in the 'mother country'. Hong Kong, for example, had wide-ranging Contagious Disease Acts and had state brothels and legalized prostitution until 1934. In other countries such as Uganda, the STD services formed the basis of the later national health services.

The Second World War and beyond

In Britain, cases of gonorrhoea were at an all time low just before the outbreak of the Second World War. Sexually transmitted diseases figured much less prominently as a social issue during this war compared with the First World War. Regulation enabled the examination and treatment of known carriers. A campaign of public education was carried out in 1942, notable for the radio appearance of the Chief Medical Officer, Sir Wilson Jameson, talking openly to the public for the first time about venereal disease.

After the war, the advent of penicillin brought a major advance in the treatment of STDs. Initial experiments in the treatment of syphilitic rabbits by the US Public Health Service in 1943 brought replication of the experiment in humans. Penicillin introduced a new era of antibiotics and the technological approach to disease that characterized medicine in the 1950s (see Chapter 12). Incidence fell dramatically in the 1950s. This meant that STDs dropped off the policy agenda in most countries and also internationally at the World Health Organization (Weindling, 1993). The coming of the contraceptive pill and its widespread availability in the UK from the 1970s through the National Heath Service brought significant changes in sexual attitudes and behaviour. Some gay men also redefined their identity based on a hedonistic sexuality. This stance was in reaction to what was seen as the outmoded medical view. In the early 1960s, rates of STDs began to climb again in many countries. In Britain, the network of treatment clinics within a speciality that had been renamed as 'genito-urinary medicine' began to offer primary health care to gay men who sought treatment for sexual infection.

The coming of HIV/AIDS

The advent of HIV (initially called GRID-Gay Related Immune Disorder) in the early 1980s emerged in many Western countries through the STD route because of the existing pattern of the utilization of services. HIV carried with it the legacy of responses to STDs. As in the late fifteenth century, there was debate about where the disease had come from. Was this an 'old disease from Africa'? Was it associated with Haitians? Or, as the British argued, was it associated with the Americans? As with STDs previously, there was debate about the appropriate policies to follow and the balance between what was good for the individual and what was good for the collective.

In many Western countries, most notably Britain and the United States, there was a strong focus on human rights, advocated by well-organized gay activist groups such as the Terrence Higgins Trust in the UK and Gay Men's Health Crisis in New York. These helped to ensure that the focus of policy was not on high-risk groups but rather on high-risk behaviours (Berridge, 1996). The international response to HIV/AIDS was also important. The role of the World Health Organization (WHO) was revived as an authoritative source of advice on STDs and more generally on health issues; a global programme on AIDS was established in 1986. AIDS was a harbinger of a new focus on globalism in health. The WHO AIDS programme was important in disseminating the focus on human rights internationally in the 1980s, and this became the dominant model for national AIDS programmes in countries of the South as well as the North. Whether this universal model was appropriate or not for all countries has been a matter of debate. Some countries, Cuba most notably, built on a different public health tradition, using confinement and isolation of HIV-infected individuals. HIV/AIDS with its initial model of rapid infection and death was a tremendous shock to the established post-war model of chronic disease, which is discussed in Chapter 12.

Exercise 6.6

The poster and voiceover below were used in the UK Government mass media campaign in 1986–1987. Look at the poster and read the voiceover before answering the questions that follow.

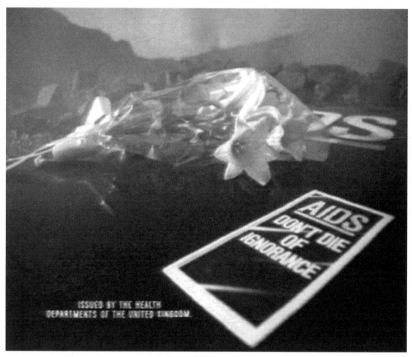

Figure 6.3 Department of Health AIDS campaign, 1986–1987

Voiceover

'There is now a danger which has become a threat to us all. It is a deadly disease and there is no known cure. The virus can be passed during sexual intercourse with an infected person. Anyone can get it, man or woman. So far it's been confined to small groups. But it's spreading. So protect yourself and read this leaflet when it arrives. If you ignore AIDS it could be the death of you. So don't die of ignorance.'

1 What is the message the poster and voiceover aim to convey?
2 At whom do you think they are directed?
3 What feelings does the poster and text convey?
4 Can you think of the significance of the date, 1986–1987?

Feedback

1 The poster and voiceover aim to convey the urgency and emergency nature of the AIDS situation and the responsibility of the population to inform themselves about

how to avoid it. The message is therefore one that is congruent with the overall focus in the recent history of public health. It is the individual's responsibility to avoid infection and the tactic to help with this is information and knowledge.

2 The campaign is directed at everyone. The poster and voiceover do not single out a particular group within the population for the message.

3 The picture and text convey feelings of gloom and fear. The imagery is of death, exemplified by the use of the lilies, common as a funeral flower.

4 The years in which this campaign took place, 1986–1987, marked the height of government and public fear that the new syndrome/disease would spread rapidly and potentially overwhelm the nation. The campaign and this image reflect that fear. It is important to remember that AIDS was incurable at this stage and death after diagnosis was rapid.

AIDS in Africa and beyond

In recent years, the focus of attention has moved from the United States and Europe to Africa and trying to understand the history of the outbreak there. The historian John Iliffe has argued that the epidemic in Africa is the worst epidemic because it was the first epidemic, and was heterosexual (Iliffe, 2006). Historians had previously focused on the crisis of syphilis in the colonies (Vaughan, 1991), as Chapter 5 mentions. But in recent years they have turned their attention to the 'pre-history' of AIDS and what led it to spread. Demographers have also asked what caused the African epidemic to take off so quickly. Some advanced explanations using theories of African sexuality and culture: African sexual norms included a culture of frequent partner exchange, and would facilitate the spread of STDs including AIDS. Such ideas have been criticized as potentially racist. Scholars are now researching the earlier history of sexual behaviour and conclude that the changes that took place in some African countries in the 1970s were significant. These included the growth of urban centres and a rise in unemployment and female poverty after the 1973 oil crisis.

There have also been debates about the histories of responses to HIV/AIDS in particular countries, especially South Africa and Uganda. In South Africa there was low fertility but high HIV prevalence, while in Uganda there was high fertility but a fall in HIV prevalence. The 'success story' in Uganda has been attributed to a policy based on abstinence, but this tactic has been disputed. The response in South Africa to HIV has also been controversial, in particular President Mbeki's opposition to the theory that HIV caused AIDS. It is easy to condemn such a stance as inexplicable, but, like other responses in history, it has to be understood in the context of its time. This was in part based on an African stance against forms of colonial imperialism – wanting to treat an African disease with African means. It sought to replace a narrow virological focus with a broader epidemiological approach that might benefit the whole population. Mbeki's stance was largely abandoned in 2002 and critics argued that his position undermined public health initiatives and led to more AIDS-related deaths (van Rijn, 2006).

The use of history

Historical work is now being used to try to understand the genesis of the African epidemic. But history was also important from the start of the epidemic. Because HIV/AIDS was a new syndrome, the only models that offered some understanding were those from history. In Britain, politicians and others turned to the past, and specifically to the history of the Contagious Diseases Acts and of venereal disease during the First World War, to try to work out appropriate strategies. In the United States the historian Allan Brandt wrote a new chapter on AIDS to add to his book on STDs (Brandt, 1987). Historians and also policy-makers were acutely aware of the historical resonance of some of the issues that AIDS brought in its train. We will return to this use of history in the final chapter of the book.

Exercise 6.7

The American historian Charles Rosenberg was among those who drew on past history to understand the response to HIV/AIDS in the present. Read the following extract from his commentary on AIDS in historical perspective and then answer the questions that follow.

> 'In many ways we have re-enacted traditional patterns of response to a perceived threat ... One of course is the gradual and grudging acceptance of the epidemic as reality ... Equally obvious is the way in which coping with randomness provides an occasion for reaffirming the social values of the majority, and for blaming victims.'
>
> (Rosenberg, 1992)

1 What are the traditional patterns of response to a perceived threat that Rosenberg mentions?
2 What does he mean by 'reaffirming the social values of the majority' in relation to HIV/AIDS?
3 Who are the victims who are blamed?

Feedback

1 The traditional pattern of response you might think of is of initial fear, but also attempts to distance oneself from possible infection through a moral interpretation of infection. Think back to the discussion of cholera in Chapter 1 and you will remember how people attributed infection to vice and moral habits as reasons for the passage of disease and whom it struck.
2 Rosenberg means that in the case of HIV/AIDS, the focus in some societies on traditional morality and the emphasis on chastity or on abstinence.
3 The victims can be groups such as gay men in some societies; or they can be what have been termed 'innocent victims', children or women who are infected by accident.

You should reflect at the end of this exercise on how HIV/AIDS has been responded to in your country over time and whether the pattern fits what Rosenberg articulates here.

Summary

The role of STDs within society has a long history. These diseases have been bound up with issues of class, gender, morality and blame. Strategies for dealing with STDs were underpinned by these wider concerns. Scientific advance took place in the early twentieth century so that causation and treatment were better understood. However, science was not the hoped for solution. It brought further dilemmas about strategies to be followed and different nations developed responses dependent on particular national factors. In more recent times, the rise of HIV/AIDS has reactivated some of the dilemmas associated with STDs and the history of responses to those diseases has been brought into policy-making. As we will see in the next chapter, attempts to control individual behaviour for the benefit of public health were rarely unproblematic.

References

Berridge V (1996) AIDS in the UK: The Making of Policy, 1981–1994. Oxford: Oxford University Press.

Brandt AM (1985) No Magic Bullet: A Social History of Venereal Disease in the United States since 1880. New York: Oxford University Press.

Brandt AM (1987) No Magic Bullet: A Social History of Venereal Disease in the United States since 1880 (revised edn). New York: Oxford University Press.

Crosby AW (1972) The Columbian Exchange: Biological and Cultural Consequences of 1492. Westport, CT: Greenwood Publishing.

Fisher K (2006) Birth Control, Sex and Marriage in Britain, 1918–1960. Oxford: Oxford University Press.

Iliffe J (2006) The African AIDS Epidemic: A History. Athens, OH: Ohio University Press/Oxford: James Currey.

Knowlton J (1832) The Fruits of Philosophy: or The Private Companion of Young Married People (published anonymously).

Lewis M and Bamber S (1997) Introduction, in Lewis M, Bamber S and Waugh M (eds) Sex, Disease and Society: A Comparative History of Sexually Transmitted Diseases and HIV/AIDS in Asia and the Pacific (pp. 1–17). Westport, CT: Greenwood Press.

Mort F (2000) Dangerous Sexualities: Medico-moral Politics in England since 1830. London: Routledge.

Rosenberg C (1992) What is an epidemic? AIDS in historical perspective, in Rosenberg C, Explaining Epidemics and Other Studies in the History of Medicine (pp. 278–292). Cambridge: Cambridge University Press.

Sauerteig L (2001) The fatherland is in danger, save the fatherland!', in Davidson R and Hall L (eds) Sex, Sin and Suffering: Venereal Disease and European Society Since 1970 (pp. 76–88). London: Routledge.

Smith FB (1990) The Contagious Diseases Acts reconsidered, Social History of Medicine, 3(2): 197–215.

Szreter S (1995) Fertility, Class and Gender in Britain, 1860–1940. Cambridge: Cambridge University Press.

Van Rijn K (2006) The politics of uncertainty: The AIDS debate, Thabo Mbeki and the South African government response, Social History of Medicine, 19(3): 521–38.

Vaughan M (1991) Curing Their Ills: Colonial Power and African Illness. Oxford: Polity Press.

Walkowitz J (1980) Prostitution and Victorian Society: Women, Class, and the State. Cambridge: Cambridge University Press.

Walkowitz J and Walkowitz D (1974) 'We are not the beasts of the field': Prostitution and the poor in Plymouth and Southampton under the Contagious Diseases Acts, in Hartman MS and Banner L (eds) Clio's Consciousness Raised: New Perspectives on the History of Women (pp. 192–225). New York: Harper & Row.

Weindling P (1993) The politics of international coordination to combat sexually transmitted disease, 1900–1980s, in Berridge V and Strong P (eds) AIDS and Contemporary History (pp. 93–107). Cambridge: Cambridge University Press.

7 | Case study: Substance use

Alex Mold

Overview

Like sexually transmitted diseases, the history of the use of psychoactive (mind-altering) substances highlights key issues about the development of public health and how it was that individual behaviours came to be seen as public health problems. In this chapter, we explore the reasons why some psychoactive substances are illegal and others are not. Different substances have been subjected to various forms of regulation throughout the past. To understand the reasons for this, drugs – and the people that used them – need to be located in historical context.

Learning objectives

After working through this chapter, you will be able to:

- describe how historical and cultural contexts shape ideas about, and responses to, the use of psychoactive substances
- use primary sources to identify and explain some of the factors that led certain substances to be defined as a problem
- distinguish between different policy responses to the use of psychoactive substances, and evaluate the reasons why these were introduced

Key terms

Addiction The notion that the compulsive use of psychoactive substances is a disease where users cannot stop taking the drug.

New public health A term used to describe changes in direction of public health from the 1970s, emphasizing a focus on disease prevention and individual behaviour as a cause of ill-health. This was a controversial development, and was linked to the parallel rise of health promotion.

Passive smoking The idea that environmental tobacco smoke poses a danger to the health of non-smokers.

Psychoactive substance A substance that has an effect on the mind when ingested orally, by inhalation or by injection.

Temperance movement An organized effort during the nineteenth century to limit, and later ban, the consumption of alcoholic drinks.

Introduction

Why is it that some psychoactive substances are illegal and others are not? Why do different systems of control exist for different substances? How have these systems changed over time? In this chapter, we will address these questions by exploring the changing fate of three types of psychoactive substance: alcohol, tobacco and what are now called illegal drugs, including opium, heroin and cocaine. Systematic attempts to control the use of these substances are a relatively recent development: up until the mid nineteenth century, alcohol, tobacco and drugs like opium were freely available and widely used. From the 1850s onwards a series of social, cultural, economic, medical and scientific factors came together to make the control of psychoactive substances seem necessary. But, these factors did not affect psychoactive substances evenly: some appeared to need stronger forms of control than others. In this chapter, we investigate why this was the case.

Exercise 7.1

Think about the current regulatory status of tobacco, alcohol, cannabis, cocaine and heroin in the country where you live. Place each substance somewhere on the line below:

Freely available to all   Restricted use, but legal for adults   Completely prohibited

←——→

Give one reason why you think each substance occupies the position allocated.

Feedback

Depending on where you live, you have probably put none of the substances at the 'freely available' end of the line, tobacco and alcohol in the middle, and cocaine and heroin at the 'completely prohibited' end of the line. However, think again about the position of alcohol. Alcohol is completely prohibited in some countries such as Saudi Arabia and Libya. Many other countries also have 'dry' regions where alcohol cannot be purchased. And, in the past, a number of countries have attempted to prohibit the use of alcohol, such as the United States from 1920 to 1933, and Russia during the early Soviet era. Other substances, such as cannabis, have moved back and forth between different points along the regulatory line. What this suggests is that psychoactive substances cannot always be placed within fixed categories; rather these change between places and over time.

Your reasons for the positioning of each substance may include factors such as:

• the danger using the substance poses to individual health
• the impact using the substance has on society
• how widely the substance is used
• vested interests (e.g. the power of the tobacco industry)

We return to this exercise at the end of the chapter to consider the *historical* reasons why substances like tobacco, alcohol and heroin have been regulated in different ways.

Alcohol

Alcohol has an ancient and global history. Viticulture, the cultivation of grapes to make wine, began between 6000 and 4000 A-B - in the region surrounding the Black Sea. The ancient Greeks and Romans knew how to turn grain and other plant extracts into spirits through distilling, a practice that spread to Europe during the eleventh century. In England, ale (beer) was widely consumed by men, women and children throughout the medieval and early modern periods, to the extent that in 1297 the Assize of Bread and Ale branded beer the 'second necessity of life'.

But, for almost as long as humans have consumed alcohol, concerns were expressed about its effects. In the Bible, Isaiah states that 'the priest and the prophet have erred through strong drink, they are swallowed up of wine' (Isaiah 28:7). In China, during the eighth century, the poet Tu Fu wrote that 'I give way to drink; I have long ceased to care that all men ignore me' (Lee, 1986). Nonetheless, in the West, concerted efforts to curb the consumption of alcohol through regulation did not really begin until the nineteenth century. Changes in the economy and society of places like Europe and North America made drinking alcohol appear more damaging than it had done in the past.

A key factor was the Industrial Revolution of the late eighteenth and early nineteenth centuries, which required a sober and orderly workforce to drive it forward. Drunk or hungover workers were a potential danger to themselves and others in an industrial environment, and worse still, so far as factory owners were concerned, they were less productive. Yet, alcohol was seen as much more than a threat to production: drink was conceived as posing a danger to social order, to public health, to morality and also individual salvation.

Exercise 7.2

Examine the Russian lithograph in Figure 7.1 entitled 'Blessed is he who does not drink wine' by T. Nemkova. Then answer this question.

• What message is the artist trying to convey about the effects of drinking alcohol?

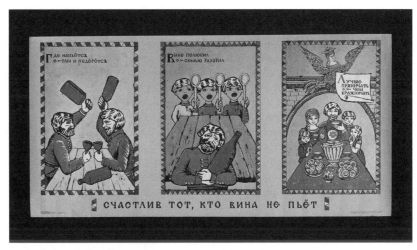

Figure 7.1 Colour lithograph by T. Nemkova, 1990
English translation of the Russian captions:
Title: 'Blessed is he who does not drink wine'
First image: 'When the gentleman gets drunk, he will become aggressive'
Second image: 'One who loved wine has destroyed his family'
Third image: 'It's better to drink tea with Lebkuchen [biscuits] than to drink alcoholic drinks'

Credit: Wellcome Library, London

Feedback

This picture is clearly designed to highlight the individual and social harm that alcohol can cause. In the first image, the two men are engaged in a drunken brawl, suggesting that the consumption of alcohol leads to violence. In the second picture, the man is shown cradling a bottle in front of his starving children. In the final image, a smiling family are shown drinking tea and eating biscuits, presumably because the man is tee-total (does not drink alcohol). Drinking alcohol, the image suggests, has consequences not just for the drinker, but also for his or her family, and by extension, for wider society too.

It may have surprised you to note that the lithograph was produced in 1990. Although the style of the image echoes anti-alcohol cartoons from the late nineteenth century, it was actually produced for a more recent campaign to limit the consumption of alcohol in the Soviet Union that began in the mid-1980s.

Controlling the consumption of alcohol

From the 1830s onwards, a series of campaigns aimed at persuading people to give up strong drink (spirits) began to take off in Britain, Europe and North America. These campaigns, known as the temperance movement, were led by middle-class social reformers, but they rapidly garnered working-class support, so that by the 1860s it was estimated that as many as one million people in Britain (out of a population of around 20 million) had taken the pledge not to drink alcohol (Harrison, 1971/1994). In the UK, temperance reformers attempted to get Parliament to prohibit alcohol completely, or failing this, to bring in much stricter controls on drink (Dingle, 1980). Although temperance reformers were ultimately unsuccessful in banning alcohol in Britain (in part because the major brewers had support within Parliament), the turn to the state was an important moment. The idea that the government should introduce legislation to control the use of alcohol was a precedent for later attempts to regulate the consumption of other psychoactive substances.

Indeed, the twentieth century saw further attempts to manage drinking. Around the time of the First World War, alcohol prohibition was introduced in eleven countries, including the United States, Russia, Norway and Canada (Schrad, 2010). After the Second World War, attention turned to the impact alcohol had on health. The idea that the compulsive consumption of alcohol was a 'disease' was not a new one (having been in circulation since at least the nineteenth century) but alcoholism was 'rediscovered' by psychiatrists in the late 1940s. In Britain, specialist treatment for alcoholics was put in place, as the disease of alcoholism was thought to be limited to a relatively small group of people (Thom and Berridge, 1995).

Some of the broader public health dimensions of drink also came into focus in the latter half of the twentieth century. The effect of alcohol on car drivers, for example, began to cause concern, a development that resulted in the introduction of the breathalyser in Britain in 1967. Research demonstrating that even fairly moderate levels of drinking could have a negative impact on health was also significant. Reducing alcohol consumption became part of more general public health initiatives such as the WHO Europe *Health For All* strategy in 1985, and the UK *Health of the Nation* strategy in 1991.

At the same time, the fears earlier expressed by the temperance movement about the effect that alcohol could have on public order and on morality remained. Media interest in 'binge drinking' in the early years of the twenty-first century suggests that many long-running anxieties surrounding drink continue to be felt. Although 'binge drinking' has been variously defined, recent representations have tended to emphasize the excessive consumption of alcoholic drinks in public places by young people. It has been argued that this focus on young drinkers, and on young women in particular, is a reflection not so much of the real extent of alcohol-related mortality, but rather an expression of long-term trends within public health where women are depicted as both 'innocent victims' and also as a 'vector of infection' (Berridge, Herring and Thom, 2009). This concept will be familiar to you from Chapter 6, where it was shown that anxiety was expressed about the impact of STDs on 'innocent victims'. Concern about alcohol use thus reflects deeper fears within society. As we will see, this is a key theme not just in the way alcohol has been dealt with, but also in the response offered to other psychoactive substances, including tobacco.

Tobacco

Compared with alcohol, tobacco is a relative newcomer, at least within European societies. Tobacco was famously brought to Europe from North America in the early modern period by explorers like Christopher Columbus and Sir Walter Raleigh. In the seventeenth century, the cultivation of tobacco by American colonists allowed for a significant growth in tobacco consumption, so that by 1670 the English were getting through an average of a pound of tobacco per head per year (Courtwright, 2001).

Yet it was not until the late nineteenth century that tobacco use became a widespread habit. The invention of the Bonsack cigarette rolling machine in 1881 brought smoking to the masses. The machine could make 300 cigarettes a minute, allowing manufacturers to reduce the price of cigarettes to within the budget of the working classes. Tobacco consumption in Europe and North America rocketed: in Britain this increased from an average of two pounds per head per year during the mid nineteenth century, to an average of seven pounds per head per year by the mid twentieth century (Hilton, 2000). In 1948, it was estimated that 82 per cent of British men smoked (Berridge, 2007).

As with alcohol, concern had long been expressed about the effects of tobacco consumption. James I of England penned a 'Counterblaste' against tobacco in 1616, but it was during the nineteenth century that an anti-tobacco movement, paralleling the temperance movement, came into being. In the UK, groups like the Anti-Tobacco Society (established in 1853) stressed the religious and medical consequences of smoking, arguing that smokers had become 'enslaved' by tobacco. Like the temperance movement, the anti-tobacco campaigners had little success in curbing tobacco consumption, but they did have some impact on restricting who could use tobacco. Anti-tobacconists played a role in the introduction of the Children's Act in Britain in 1908, which made it illegal to sell tobacco to anyone under the age of sixteen.

The idea that tobacco smoking could pose a danger to health was clearly not a new one, but in the 1950s new evidence, and new ways of viewing this, came into being. Epidemiological research carried out by Richard Doll and Sir Austin Bradford Hill (who were based at the London School of Hygiene and Tropical Medicine) was to prove crucial in establishing a link between smoking and lung cancer. In a now famous article published in the *British Medical Journal* in 1950, Doll and Hill suggested that smoking was an important factor in the production of carcinoma of the lung (Doll and Hill, 1950). Later studies confirmed the statistical association between smoking and lung cancer, as well as also other conditions, such as coronary heart disease. Yet, Doll and Hill's message was not universally accepted at the time: other potential causes of cancer of the lung, such as air pollution, were also considered. Moreover, accepting Doll and Hill's findings also required the recognition of the validity of risk factor epidemiology, which was a relatively new way of viewing the causation of disease at the time (Berridge, 2007).

By the early 1960s, the medical profession and health policy-makers appeared to have reached a consensus on the dangers of smoking for health, but translating this into public health policy was to prove challenging.

Exercise 7.3

Read the extract below, which is taken from the UK Royal College of Physicians 1962 report, *Smoking and Health*. Then answer the questions that follow.

'Preventive Measures

Since it is not yet possible to identify those individuals who will be harmed by smoking, preventive measures must be generally applied.

The harmful effects of cigarette smoking might be reduced by efficient filters, by using modified tobaccos, by leaving longer cigarette stubs or by changing from cigarette to pipe or cigar smoking.

General discouragement of smoking, particularly by young people, is necessary. More effort needs to be expended on discovering the most effective means of dissuading children from starting the smoking habit.

There can be no doubt of our responsibility for protecting future generations from developing the dependence on cigarette smoking that is so widespread today.

Most adults have heard of the risks of cigarette smoking but remain unconvinced. Doctors, who see the consequences of the habit, have reduced their cigarette consumption. Some evidence of concern by the Government is needed to convince the public. The Government have so far only asked local health authorities to carry out health education in respect of smoking, but little seems to have been achieved. The Central Council for Health Education and Local Authorities spent less than £5,000 on anti-smoking education in 1956–60, while the Tobacco Manufacturers spent £38,000,000 on advertising their goods during this period.'

Extract from Royal College of Physicians (1962)

1 List the key measures recommended by the report to prevent the harmful effects of smoking.
2 What barriers might have existed to the successful implementation of such measures?

Feedback

1 The report emphasizes a series of preventive measures to limit the dangers posed by smoking. These include:

- developing less harmful cigarettes
- changing smoking behaviour to smoke more safely
- discouraging people, particularly children, from starting smoking
- convincing smokers to reduce their cigarette consumption through a public information campaign

2 The report also hints at a number of possible barriers to the successful implementation of such measures. You may have noted down factors such as:

- technical difficulties in developing safer smoking materials
- problems with effecting behavioural change: how do you discourage people from starting to smoke, or encourage people to smoke more safely, or to reduce their consumption?
- problems with communicating the anti-smoking message, such as a lack of resources to pay for anti-smoking campaigns, and the relative power and wealth of the tobacco industry

As the extract from the *Smoking and Health* report suggests, in the UK some effort did go in to the development of safer smoking materials in the 1960s. But, by the 1970s, emphasis had shifted away from reducing the harm associated with smoking, and towards encouraging people to give up the habit altogether. This shift was representative of broader changes within public health. Individual behaviour and lifestyle choices (like smoking) came to be seen as important factors in disease causation. The so-called 'new public health', which emerged in the 1970s, emphasized the risks to health that certain behaviours posed. We return to the 'new public health' in more detail in Chapter 12, but its significance here is that it encouraged a focus on changing the behaviour of individuals, in this case getting people to stop smoking. Such a move placed renewed emphasis on personal responsibility for health, a development that could have the consequence of blaming sick individuals for their condition.

Indeed, in many countries in the developed world, smoking has become an increasingly stigmatized activity, something reflected in, and exacerbated by, the changing demographic profile of smokers. In Britain, from the mid-1970s onwards, smoking rates began to fall, although not evenly across socio-economic categories. As Table 7.1 shows, the number of British men and women who smoked fell between 1948 and 2008.

Table 7.1 The percentage of men and women aged 16 and over who smoked in Britain, 1948–2008

| Year | Prevalence of smoking | |
	Males (%)	Females (%)
1948	65	41
1953	59	37
1958	58	39
1963	54	43
1968	55	43
1974	51	41
1979	43	36
1985	36	32
1991	30	28
1996	29	26
2002	27	25
2008	22	21

Source: Post-1974, Office for National Statistics, 2009; pre-1974, Wald and Nicholaides-Bourman, 1991.

The middle classes gave up smoking much more rapidly than the working classes, so that by 2004, it was estimated that 33 per cent of men and 30 per cent of women in manual occupations smoked, compared with 20 per cent of men and 17 per cent of women in managerial occupations (General Household Survey, quoted in Berridge, 2007). The changing pattern of who smoked made it easier to mount a more aggressive campaign against smoking and smokers, as the habit was increasingly associated with the poor (Berridge, 1999a).

The marginalization of smokers was further exacerbated by the emergence of passive smoking as a public health concern. In the early 1980s, a study was published which showed that the non-smoking wives of heavy smokers had a much higher risk of developing lung cancer (Hirayama, 1981). Later work appeared to confirm this, and exposure to environmental tobacco smoke, or passive smoking, became a key public health issue. What was also significant about the emergence of passive smoking was that it led to additional changes in the way in which the threat posed by tobacco was seen. Through exposure to tobacco smoke by 'passive' or 'involuntary' smoking, the health of the general population, not just smokers, appeared to be endangered. The threat to others raised by passive smoking, particularly to so-called 'innocent victims' such as women (as the wives of male smokers) and children, helped drive forward more restrictive measures against tobacco in some countries. Banning smoking in public places in the UK and elsewhere became a practical policy option, which it had not previously been (Berridge, 1999a). The danger to others posed by tobacco had come to play a role in the regulation of this substance, just as it did for alcohol, and as we will see in the next section, it was important for other psychoactive drugs too.

Illegal drugs

All of the psychoactive substances that are prohibited today, including drugs like heroin, cocaine, cannabis and amphetamines, began their histories as legally used products. Attempts to ban the use of these drugs only really began in the twentieth century: before then many now prohibited substances were widely used and subjected to few controls. Like alcohol and tobacco, the use of illegal drugs has a long history. Opium, for example, may have been the first psychoactive substance ever taken by early humans, even before alcohol, as it does not require fermentation or distillation to be used. Cultivated opium poppy seeds have been found at Neolithic (Stone Age) sites in Switzerland, and in Mesopotamia (modern-day Iraq) (Booth, 1996).

During the sixteenth century, exploration opened up the potential for an international trade in psychoactive substances on an unprecedented scale. Although opium had been an important part of Western medicine for centuries, the development of laudanum (opium dissolved in alcohol) by the English physician Thomas Sydenham in the 1660s helped to facilitate the use of opium as a cure-all for a vast range of illnesses, from constipation to gout. Self-medication with opium became commonplace in Europe and North America: by 1827 the English were consuming over a pound of opium per thousand people a year, and by 1860 this had risen to over three pounds of opium per thousand people annually (Berridge, 1999b).

Despite the widespread use of opium in Britain and other countries for what might be termed medical and non-medical purposes, it was not until the second half of the nineteenth century that this was seen as particularly problematic. During this period a series of factors combined to make the use of opium, and other psychoactive substances like alcohol and tobacco, appear more dangerous.

First, technical and economic developments brought with them greater potential for problematic drug use. More potent forms of drugs, such as morphine and heroin, began to appear from the 1820s onwards. At the same time, a more effective mechanism for drug delivery was becoming available, through the invention of the hypodermic syringe in 1856. Newer drugs like morphine and heroin could also be mass produced and sold on a commercial basis. This meant that more people were able to use stronger drugs in a more efficient way, which raised the possibility of more harmful drug use.

Second, perceptions of drug use started to change during the nineteenth century. As we have seen with alcohol and tobacco, the wider implications of psychoactive drug use came to the attention of reformers. The temperance movement, with its emphasis on the moral, religious and social harm that alcohol could cause, helped to alter the way psychoactive substance use was viewed. Widespread opiate taking came to be regarded as a potential danger to public health. In Britain and other countries, particular concern was expressed about the practice of giving babies and small children soothing syrups that contained opium, a practice known as 'infant-doping' (Berridge, 1999b).

Third, developments in pharmacy and in medicine brought psychoactive substance use to the attention of the medical profession. As the status and power of medicine and pharmacy grew in this period (see Chapter 4), doctors and pharmacists began to demand more control over the drugs they administered and those who used them. Systems for pharmaceutical regulation, such as the British Pharmacy Act of 1868, limited the sale of opiates and other poisons to pharmacies and demanded that those buying the drug sign a register stating that they knew they were purchasing a potentially dangerous substance. Meanwhile, doctors began to see the compulsive use of opiates (and other drugs, including alcohol) as a discrete disease, a condition they called addiction.

Finally, fear of drugs, and more importantly of the people that were thought to be using them, played a role in shaping demands for greater drug control. Drug use in the late nineteenth and early twentieth centuries was often associated with marginalized populations. In Britain, opium smoking was believed to be rife among Chinese immigrants. Once again, the perceived threat psychoactive substance use posed to innocent victims was stressed, in this case that evil Chinese men would 'dope' innocent white women to have sex with them. In the United States, cocaine use was widely associated with African-Americans, and similar fears were expressed about the threat these 'coke fiends' posed to white women. What is significant is that the concerns voiced about minority drug taking did not reflect actual patterns of use in this period, but were rather a manifestation of deeper fears about immigration, race, gender and sexuality (Kohn, 1992).

Exercise 7.4

Read the three extracts below, which are taken from newspaper articles published in the *Daily Express* and the *Daily Mail* in December 1918. Then answer the questions that follow.

Extract 1

'The government restrictions on the sale of cocaine are as stringent as it is possible to make them ... Where, then, do the people who carry out the traffic obtain cocaine?

The answer is: from the Chinese in Limehouse [area in East London, close to the docks]. Nearly all the cocaine sold in the West End [of London] is smuggled into this country. Before it gets into the hands, or rather the arm, of the actual "dope fiend" quite a number of persons have made a substantial profit, but traced back to its source it comes from Chinatown nearly every time, the Chinatown of Thomas Burke [author of a collection of sensational accounts of life amongst Chinese immigrants] that is as unfamiliar to the average Londoner as Tibet, despite the fact that it is only some three miles from Piccadilly-circus.'

Taken from the *Daily Express*, 17 December 1918, p. 1

Extract 2

'Doctors, heads of institutions, and social workers agree that "doping" is not a deliberate vice. Rather it is a fashionable habit, an artificial war product, which will disappear with the return of more normal conditions. It is a vice of the neurotic, not of the normal. "Men" said a specialist, "do not as a rule take to drugs unless there is a hereditary influence, but women are more temperamentally attracted".'

Taken from the *Daily Mail*, 16 December 1918

Extract 3

'One of the most terrible aspects of the drug traffic in London is the way in which men and women, and even young girls, who have led clean, sane and healthy lives, are induced by drug fiends to take the first steps that lead to the underworld ...

...The young actress or artist may easily get in touch with genuinely vicious and decadent people without realising that she is slipping on the wrong side of the border-line.

Girls new to the life and innocent of the lures of the underworld meet these absorbingly interesting and apparently wealthy bohemians. Moral infection takes place. They take a pipe or two of opium or a sniff of cocaine – and they like the adventure. The next time they are dull or bored they naturally turn to it again.'

Taken from the *Daily Express*, 9 December 1918, p. 1

1 Who, according to Extract 1, is responsible for the illegal drug trade? Why do you think this group is being picked out?
2 Who, according to Extract 2, are the main victims of drug use? Why do you think this group is being picked out?
3 Comment on the impression given in Extract 3 about the effects of drug use. What do you think the extract is suggesting might happen to drug takers?

Feedback

1 You may have noticed that Extract 1 refers to new regulations to control the sale of drugs under the Defence of the Realm Act 1916. In the absence of a legal supply of drugs, the article suggests that the Chinese have begun trading in drugs illegally. Once again, it is important to stress that this was not a reflection so much of the actual pattern of drug use at the time, but rather an attempt to hold an already stigmatized population responsible for the spread of illegal drug use.
2 Although Extract 2 mentions both male and female drug users it is quite clear that women are thought to be most vulnerable to the effects of cocaine. Note that the article suggests women are 'temperamentally attracted' to cocaine, as are 'neur-otics'. This fits with the contemporary view that women were more likely to suffer from 'nervous disorders', what we might today term mental illness. Fears about the effect drug use had on women were related to longer running concerns about their sexual behaviour, and also their fitness to be wives and mothers. These fears were similar to those discussed in Chapter 6, where we looked at ideas about the spread of sexually transmitted disease.
3 Extract 3 expresses the view that normally 'clean, sane, and healthy' people, especially young women, are exposed to moral danger through drug use. Drug taking brings them into contact with 'genuinely vicious and decadent people' and 'moral infection' takes place. This seems to be implying that drug use is morally bad and that it may lead to other kinds of immoral behaviour, perhaps of a sexual nature. Again, note that the focus is very much on the harm drugs can do to young women: as with alcohol and tobacco attention was often paid to the 'innocent victims' of psychoactive substance use.

Controlling illegal drugs

During and immediately after the First World War, fears about drug use resulted in the introduction of legislation to control psychoactive substances both nationally and internationally. New systems of regulation appeared to be required to deal with the threat to health, morality and society that certain drugs posed. In the UK, wartime restrictions limiting the sale of drugs like morphine and cocaine to those with a prescription were extended through the Dangerous Drugs Act in 1920. In the United States, the Harrison Narcotic Act of 1914 prohibited the prescription of 'narcotic' drugs to individuals addicted to these, and made addiction to drugs like heroin a criminal offence. At the same time, global restrictions on the trade in illegal drugs were also introduced. International meetings in Shanghai in 1909, and in The Hague in 1911–1912, 1913 and 1914 recommended that the trade in drugs should be confined to those used only for 'legitimate medical purposes'. Following the First World War, the Versailles Treaty entrusted the League of Nations with the control of the trade in dangerous drugs, a responsibility taken over by the United Nations after the Second World War. In 1961, the Single Convention on Narcotic Drugs was introduced, prohibiting trade in drugs like heroin, cannabis and cocaine, and requiring signatory countries to implement domestic law to ban the use of these substances.

Yet, the legal restrictions introduced to regulate psychoactive substance use were not the only way in which illegal drugs were controlled in the twentieth century: running alongside the legal system were forms of medical control. In Britain, drugs such as heroin and cocaine could be legally used if prescribed by a doctor to his or her patient. Indeed, this was allowed even if the patient was addicted to the drug concerned. This was the so-called 'British System', which permitted doctors to prescribe drugs to addicts on a long-term – or maintenance – basis, if all attempts to withdraw from the drug had failed. Such an approach contrasted with methods of treatment elsewhere in the world: in the United States, for example, heroin prescription was completely prohibited, even for the relief of severe pain.

It is generally agreed that the 'British System' was allowed because the number of known drug addicts was small, and addicts were usually middle-aged, middle class and had usually become addicted to morphine or heroin as a result of treatment for another condition (Berridge, 1999b). But, as the addict population began to change, so too did the stringency of medical regulation of both drugs and users. By the 1960s, addicts were younger, and had usually begun taking drugs for recreational reasons. More severe measures of control seemed to be required, including the introduction of specialist treatment centres for heroin addiction, restrictions on who could prescribe heroin to addicts, and the notification of addiction to a central authority, as with infectious diseases. Drug addiction was being seen as a public health problem: heroin use was thought to affect not just the user, but also the wider community in which he or she lived (Mold, 2008).

To rid the community of this danger, different approaches were pursued. During the 1970s and early 1980s, many doctors involved in the treatment of addiction focused on getting users off drugs, often by prescribing the substitute methadone on a reducing basis. The appearance of HIV/AIDS among injecting drug users forced something of a change in policy in the second half of the 1980s, with emphasis being placed on preventing drug users from spreading HIV by sharing needles, and other harm reduction methods (Berridge, 1996).

Notwithstanding the clear public health imperatives associated with drug use, legal measures to control drugs, and those who used them, continued. Indeed, by the 1990s and 2000s, legal and medical approaches to drug use seemed to be coming together with the introduction of measures such as Drug Treatment and Testing Orders, which referred individuals convicted on drug offences to treatment instead of prison. Although psychoactive substances such as heroin look likely to remain illegal in most countries, legal methods of control exist alongside, and are often intertwined with, public health approaches to drug use.

Why are drugs legal or illegal?

As we have seen, different psychoactive substances have been subjected to different systems of control throughout history, but some drugs have been completely prohibited. Why is this? Perhaps it is the case that, over time, the most harmful drugs have been subjected to stricter forms of control? Or, have other factors played a role too?

Exercise 7.5

In 2007, a group of researchers led by the neuropsychopharmacologist David Nutt, attempted to develop a rational scale to assess the harm that drugs cause. The researchers asked other drug experts to rank how harmful a particular substance was by using a nine-category matrix that listed a set of harms known to be associated with drug use.

Take a look at Table 7.2, which reproduces the harm matrix used by Nutt and his colleagues. Next, examine Figure 7.2, which shows the mean harm scores for twenty substances ranked by experts according to the harm matrix. Then answer the questions that follow.

Table 7.2 The harm matrix

Type of harm	Specific effects
Physical harm	Acute
	Chronic
	Intravenous harm
Dependence	Intensity of pleasure
	Psychological dependence
	Physical dependence
Social harms	Intoxication
	Other social harms
	Health-care costs

Source: Adapted from Nutt et al. (2007)

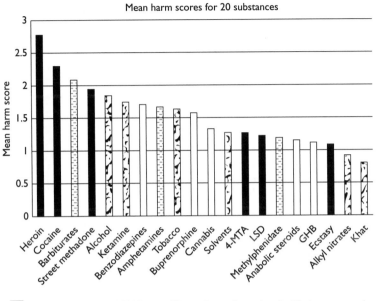

Class A: Illegal under UK Misuse of Drugs Act and associated with the strongest legal penalties, including up to 7 years imprisonment and/or an unlimited fine for possession

Class B: Illegal under UK Misuse of Drugs Act and associated with strong legal penalties, including up to 5 years imprisonment and/or an unlimited fine for possession

Class C: Illegal under UK Misuse of Drugs Act and associated with moderate legal penalties, including up to 2 years imprisonment and/or an unlimited fine for possession

No class: Legally available, although there may be some restrictions on sale and use

Figure 7.2 Mean harm scores for twenty substances

Source: Adapted from Nutt et al. (2007

1 What, according to Nutt and colleagues are the five most harmful drugs?
2 Does anything surprise you about the order in which the twenty drugs are listed?
3 What conclusions can you draw about the relationship between the harm associated with a drug and its legal status?

Feedback

1 The five most harmful drugs according to Nutt and colleagues are: (1) heroin, (2) cocaine, (3) barbiturates, (4) street methadone and (5) alcohol.
2 Given the legal status of alcohol in the UK, you may have been surprised to find alcohol in the top five most dangerous drugs. You may also not have expected to see that other legally available drugs, like tobacco, were considered to be more harmful than Class A illegal drugs, like LSD and ecstasy.

3   If we accept Nutt and his colleagues' findings, it is clear that the harm associated
    with a psychoactive substance is not necessarily related to its legal status, as
    comparatively harmful drugs like alcohol are legal and comparatively less harmful
    substances, such as ecstasy, are illegal. But, to what extent can the harms associated
    with psychoactive substances be assessed rationally, even today?

The reasons why certain psychoactive substances are legal and others are not is not
directly connected to any objective sense of the harm these cause, even if this were
possible to define. Alcohol and tobacco kill millions of people a year, and yet in most
countries they remain legal, if restricted, substances. Why?

The persistence of psychoactive substance use

Think back to the extract from the *Smoking and Health* report we examined in
Exercise 7.3. The report listed a number of reasons why it might be hard to prevent
some of the dangers posed by smoking, such as the difficulty of changing individual
behaviour, and the power and influence of the tobacco industry. Both of these factors
have played a role in tobacco's continued legality, and the same could be said for
alcohol.

Alcohol and tobacco began to be consumed on a mass scale in the nineteenth and
early twentieth centuries. By the 2000s, 90 per cent of British men and 86 per cent of
British women drank alcohol; and around a quarter of British people smoked.
Furthermore, alcohol and tobacco have long been used by cultural and political elites
– think of Winston Churchill and his cigar, or the willingness of more recent politicians,
like US President Barack Obama, to be pictured drinking beer with supporters. Not
only are elite figures unlikely to ban something that they themselves enjoy, the ubiquity
of drink, and to a lesser extent tobacco, confirms the cultural significance attached to
these substances.

In addition to the social and cultural importance of alcohol and tobacco, these substances were economically significant too. In early twentieth century Russia, it was
estimated that the tax raised from alcohol was equal to the entire military budget
(Courtwright, 2001). The large revenues generated from alcohol mean that the alcoholic drinks industry has been able to exert some influence in the corridors of power:
remember the attempt to prohibit alcohol in nineteenth-century Britain? Legislation to
ban alcohol was not passed by Parliament because MPs (Members of Parliament) with
connections to the brewing industry would not vote for the Bill.

If these factors help to explain why alcohol and tobacco remain legal, why are other
drugs like cocaine and cannabis illegal? Think back to some of the examples considered
earlier in the chapter. Recall that the drug use that was seen as the most harmful in the
past was often associated with marginalized groups such as ethnic minorities. Drug use
tended to be seen as less harmful when it was associated with more established groups,
as with the middle-aged, middle-class heroin users of the 1920s.

This is still the case today. For example, in the United States, trafficking crack cocaine
(a drug often associated with poor, black users) attracts much stiffer legal penalties
than trafficking the same amount of powder cocaine (more often associated with affluent, white users). What this suggests is that even if it is possible to scientifically determine the harm a drug can cause, it is impossible to separate the drug out from the
social, cultural and historical context in which it is used.

Exercise 7.6

Let us now return to the exercise you attempted at the beginning of the chapter. Repeat the same first step of the exercise: think about the current regulatory status of tobacco, alcohol, cannabis, cocaine and heroin in the country where you live. Place each substance somewhere on the line below:

Freely available   Restricted use, but legal for adults   Completely prohibited

What *historical* reasons are there for tobacco, alcohol, cannabis, cocaine and opium to occupy the positions you have given them?

Feedback

Although it will depend on where you live, and the restrictions imposed in your country on psychoactive substance use, your reasons for placing psychoactive substances like alcohol and tobacco in the restricted use category might include:

- used by large sections of the population, including political elites
- social and cultural significance
- economic importance
- power of drink/tobacco industry

And your reasons for placing substances like cocaine and opium in the completely prohibited category might include:

- small scale of use
- association with stigmatized groups, such as ethnic minorities (you will recall that in the nineteenth century opium was associated with the Chinese in Britain and cocaine in America with African-Americans) and women (as seen in the newspaper extracts).

Summary

The use of psychoactive substances has an ancient and global history. For centuries, people throughout the world have used different types of drugs. In the West during the nineteenth century, economic, technical, social and medical factors made the use of certain substances appear to be problematic. Regulations to control tobacco and alcohol were introduced during the early twentieth century, but other psychoactive drugs were completely banned in this period. The reasons for this related as much to who was using these substances as to the 'real' harm they caused. The mass consumption of alcohol and tobacco – and the use of these substances by powerful elites – made long-term prohibition unlikely in many countries. On the other hand, the use of psychoactive drugs such as opium and cocaine tended to be associated with stigmatized groups, allowing more restrictive legislation to be passed. To explain the current regulation of all psychoactive substances, it is therefore necessary to understand their history so that they can be placed in proper social, cultural and economic context.

References and further reading

Berridge V (1996) *AIDS in the UK: The Making of Policy, 1981–1994*. Oxford: Oxford University Press.

Berridge V (1999a) Passive smoking and its pre-history in Britain: policy speaks to science?, *Social Science and Medicine*, 49: 1183–95.

Berridge V (1999b) *Opium and the People: Opiate Use and Drug Control Policy in Nineteenth Century and Early Twentieth Century England*. London: Free Association Books.

Berridge V (2007) *Marketing Health: Smoking and the Discourse of Public Health in Britain, 1945–2000*. Oxford: Oxford University Press.

Berridge V, Herring R and Thom B (2009) Binge drinking: A confused concept and its contemporary history, *Social History of Medicine*, 22(3): 597–607.

Booth M (1996) *Opium: A Short History*. London: Simon & Schuster.

Courtwright DT (2001) *Forces of Habit: Drugs and the Making of the Modern World*. Cambridge, MA: Harvard University Press.

Dingle AE (1980) *The Campaign for Prohibition in Victorian England: The United Kingdom Alliance 1872–1895*. London: Croom Helm.

Doll R and Hill AB (1950) Smoking and carcinoma of the lung: Preliminary report, *British Medical Journal*, 30: 739–48.

Harrison B (1971/1994) *Drink and the Victorians: The Temperance Question in England, 1815–1872*. London: Faber & Faber.

Hilton M (2000) *Smoking in British Popular Culture, 1800–2000*. Manchester: Manchester University Press.

Hirayama T (1981) Non-smoking wives of heavy smokers have a higher risk of lung cancer: A study from Japan, *British Medical Journal*, 282: 183–5.

Kohn M (1992) *Dope Girls: The Birth of the British Drug Underground*. London: Granta.

Lee J (1986) Alcohol in Chinese poems: References to drunkenness, flushing and drinking. *Contemporary Drug Problems*, 13: 303–38.

Mold A (2008) *Heroin: The Treatment of Addiction in Twentieth Century Britain*. De Kalb, IL: Northern Illinois University Press.

Nutt D, King L, Saulsbury W and Blakemore C (2007) The development of a rational scale to assess the harm of drugs of potential misuse, *The Lancet*, 369: 1047–53.

Office for National Statistics (2009) *General Household Survey, 2009*. London: ONS.

Royal College of Physicians (1962) *Smoking and Health*. London: Pitman.

Schrad M (2010) *The Political Power of Bad Ideas: Networks, Institutions and the Global Prohibition Wave*. Oxford: Oxford University Press.

Thom B and Berridge V (1995) 'Special units for common problems': The birth of alcohol treatment units in England, *Social History of Medicine*, 8: 75–93.

Wald N and Nicholaides-Bourman A (1991) *UK Smoking Statistics*. Oxford: Oxford University Press.

Case study: Malaria

8

Maureen Malowany and Suzanne Taylor

Overview

This chapter offers a different sort of case study to those detailed in previous chapters: here we consider the changing public health response to a specific disease, but in a variety of different contexts. In this chapter, we explore the history of malaria and its control in Italy and Africa over the past 100 years. Although malaria has become an important target of research and global public health interventions, the disease remains a public health challenge. We will highlight the complexity of this challenge as we explore attempts, successful and unsuccessful, to control or eradicate malaria over the past 100 years. What has worked in the past – what can we learn for the present and future?

Learning objectives

After working through this chapter, you will be able to:

- explain the complexity of the transmission cycle of malaria
- identify the periods of developments in malaria control, eradication and elimination – goals, tools, strategies
- identify the epidemiological challenges for specific malarial regions
- assess the strategies of contemporary global health interventions

Key terms

Endemicity The degree to which malaria was thought to be endemic (constantly present in the population). This varied considerably over time and place: a key factor in understanding malaria control is the prevalence and periodicity of malaria transmission.

Malaria control Reducing the disease burden to a level at which it is no longer a public health problem.

Malaria elimination Interrupting local mosquito-borne malaria transmission in a defined geographical area; imported cases will continue to occur.

Malaria eradication Permanent reduction to zero of the worldwide incidence of malaria.

Plasmodia The malaria parasite. The two most common are *Plasmodium falciparum* and *Plasmodium vivax*.

Introduction

Interest in malaria holds a formidable place in global public health. In the twenty-first century, this concern is articulated through journals dedicated to malaria research, multiple international global health donors including the Gates Foundation and the Global Fund, regional partners (Multilateral Initiative for Malaria) and international research collaborations (Malaria Eradication Research Agenda – malERA). The malaria research community includes multiple disciplines and methodologies – epidemiologists, medical anthropologists, entomologists, immunologists, health systems modellers and economists, geographic/demographic spatial modellers. Although our malaria knowledge base has grown with the development of new tools and methodologies, the problem of malaria control, eradication or elimination rests with the particular combination of human populations, parasites and vectors cohabiting in a shared environment. Changes in any one aspect of this malaria-producing landscape affect all others. The epidemiological challenge is to understand all interactions within this shared environment: the human body, the mosquito vector and the parasite.

In this chapter, as we explore the discoveries, campaigns and interventions of the past 100 years, we need to ask about those puzzle pieces not addressed by any single response to the malaria challenge. There have been successes and failures. We need to learn from both.

Exercise 8.1

Examine the map below produced by the Malaria Elimination Group in 2011. What does the map tell you about the relationship between development and attempts to control malaria, both successful and unsuccessful?

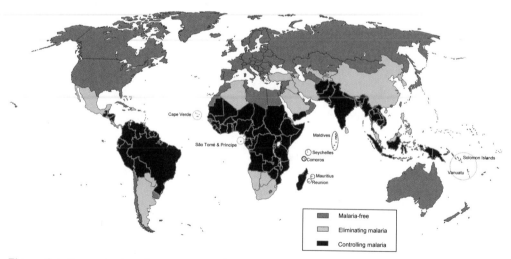

Figure 8.1 Categorization of countries as malaria-free, eliminating malaria or controlling malaria, 2012

Source: http://www.malariaeliminationgroup.org/resources/elimination-countries (accessed on 29 July 2011)

Feedback

The map shows areas that are malaria-free (where malaria has been eradicated or where malaria does not exist) or where the process of elimination or control is being undertaken. Strategies to reduce the burden of malaria have varied over time and place. The map indicates a positive relationship between socio-economic development and reduction of malaria as a disease burden. The less developed areas carry the highest burden of malaria. As of 2010, malaria-free areas have been achieved but elimination has not been achieved anywhere. Note the use of terminology. Do you understand the different terms? In this case, the phrase malaria-free has been introduced to replace the term 'eradicated' and has been applied to areas that have never had malaria. Some areas that are deemed malaria-free may face the possibility of re-emergence.

Malaria: The disease – from miasma to vectors

Fevers have been reported since ancient times, as early as the writings of Hippocrates in the fourth century A-B. Until the early twentieth century, fevers were believed to be caused by 'bad air', noxious fumes coming from foul-smelling swamps. Indeed, from 'bad air' comes the term 'mal-aria'. As we saw in Chapter 3, the theory of 'miasma' assumed that 'place' and 'space' were the important determinants of good health or disease. In the UK and Europe, populations believed that smelly marshes or putrid waters caused malaria – a fever that could lead to death. All was to change in the late nineteenth century, as scientists discovered the malaria transmission cycle. The cycle is incredibly complex and brings together a parasite, a mosquito vector and human populations. There is also dispute about which scientific contributions were most responsible for the elucidation of malaria transmission. Malaria parasites were identified in a soldier's blood in 1890 by Dr Alphonse Laveran. Other doctors and scientists studying or treating malaria checked blood for parasite presence as indicators of the presence of the 'disease'. These parasites were named 'plasmodia' by Italian scientists. But it was the English researcher Ronald Ross who established the vector link – that it was the mosquito that carried the parasite – and made the mosquito central to the transmission cycle. In 1902, Ross won the Nobel Prize for Medicine for this discovery.

Exercise 8.2

Study this extract below from an article by the physician Sir Patrick Manson regarding the emerging research on the transmission of malaria. Manson had already hypothesized that a parasite carried by mosquitoes was involved in the transmission of malaria, but it was Ross that correctly identified the parasite within the *Anopheles* mosquito in 1897. Once you have read the extract, answer the questions that follow.

'Although no argument or fact of importance has been advanced against the mosquito-malaria theory, and although it has been approved by some writers of standing, it has nevertheless been looked on askance by not a few. I have been stigmatised as a sort of pathological Jules Verne, and hinted at as being governed by "speculative considerations" and as being "guided by the divining rod of preconceived idea". It seemed to me that the theory I enunciated was the logical outcome of well ascertained facts, and the most likely explanation of the relationship of these facts to each other, and the most promising guide to fresh facts. Despite my critics, I still think that work undertaken with the object of advancing knowledge is most economically expended if directed by "speculative consideration" and "preconceived idea", provided these considerations and ideas are founded on facts, and are compatible with ascertained facts.

The speculation in question has certainly guided Ross to further and important facts, all of which point to the conclusion I ventured to indicate. After three years of incessant labour on the mosquito theory, Ross firmly believes in it, and, if I may be allowed to say so, there is no one with a better right to form, or more capable of forming, a sound opinion on the matter. My object in making this communication is three-fold. First, again to call the attention of workers on malaria to this promising field for investigation; secondly, to place on record Ross's claims to priority in discovery; and, lastly, to vindicate myself from the charge of unscientific and unwarrantable speculation'.

Manson (1898, p. 1575)

1 What does the extract imply about how Ross's theory was received?
2 What do you think this change in knowledge would mean for public health responses to malaria?

Feedback

1 The source suggests that Ross's theory was not initially widely accepted. Responsibility for the discovery and the significance of Ross's work was controversial and his findings were contested by Italian and French malariologists. Bignami, for example, had argued that mosquitoes transmitted malaria to humans in 1896 and worked with Grassi to attempt to demonstrate this. Grassi went on to indicate the role of the *Anopheles* mosquito specifically. The theory left numerous questions unanswered: Why was malaria found where the *Anopheles* was scarce especially the case in Europe? Other theories abounded, for example, the concept that malaria was a water-borne disease continued in some circles. Ross and Manson pressed for recognition and Ross received the Nobel Prize in 1902.

2 Ross's research demonstrating that the mosquito carried malaria opened the door to malaria control that focused on mosquito reduction and the development of eradication programmes. His theory gained acceptance in British colonial medicine in the context of imperial expansion. Malaria hindered economic development and engendered fear of 'the white man's grave'. The new theory indicated weak points in the transmission cycle and made it practical for public health officials to eradicate the disease. Removing the breeding grounds of the mosquito – swamps, marshes, free standing water – was a way of breaking the cycle of infection. Getting rid of the mosquito or preventing bites would prevent malaria. However, at this time there were no long-acting insecticides, or cheap, effective anti-malaria prophylactics.

The transmission cycle

Mosquitoes develop in multiple settings or situations – some only in water, others only in shade, while others can breed and develop in full sunlight. Mosquito control equals breeding control: thus targets are either at the larval or adult stage. Entomologists therefore play a crucial role in providing mosquito identification and behaviour knowledge crucial to facilitate mosquito control.

Once transmitted to the human body by the mosquito, the parasite undergoes two developmental phases. Thus although the vector's role was understood by the early twentieth century, it would take another fifty years and contributions from many other researchers in parasitology, molecular biology and immunology to describe the parasite's developmental cycles. These complexities are the foundation of the challenges for developing effective malaria prophylaxis and treatment in humans.

Malaria control

Once the transmission cycle had been explained, the next step was to tackle the disease. In the popular press, the miasma theory remained dominant until the 1920s. Among malariologists, however, there was a growing consensus on the transmission cycle itself. The question on which malariologists disagreed was how to manage or control malaria. The first of many debates emerged as to where in the transmission cycle an intervention would be most effective. Angelo Celli's contribution was significant to this discussion. Looking back in time to malaria challenges in Europe, he stated that economic development was responsible for clearing malarious areas in Europe. He pointed to his own country, Italy, demonstrating how the developed north was rid of malaria while the less developed south retained malarious areas. As a public health official, he was concerned with population-level health and advocated better agricultural methods that would include swamp drainage and social reform (Packard, 2007). Malaria control and eradication through a combination of environmental engineering and socio-economic development became one of the primary strategic arms of the twentieth-century malaria eradication movement.

Strategies and tools I: 1900–1940 – the Italian case

Ronald Ross' strategies targeted the vector, with the aim of controlling mosquito breeding at the larval stage. Reducing the number of mosquitoes would result in fewer infected mosquitoes and thus reduced malaria morbidity and mortality in human populations. Ross believed that 'Mosquito Brigades' were necessary to eliminate mosquito larvae from stagnant pools and marshes and so advised the British government to such effect before the First World War (Bynum, 1999; Dobson, 1999; Fantini, 1999). These new methods of control built upon the Italian scientists' and Ross's contributions. Control was two- pronged. First, the vector was targeted at the larval stage, through the clearance of marshes and free-standing water, which reduced the insect population. Second, human protection from mosquitoes was promoted by limiting the opportunities to be bitten by infected insects. Italy understood malaria to be an economic burden and took up this challenge with vigour.

Exercise 8.3

Examine the cartoon below from around 1900 by Amedeo John Engel Terzi (1872–1956), an Italian illustrator showing three members of the Roman Campagna Malaria Commission carrying their equipment. Terzi joined two tropical disease researchers, Louis Sambon and George Carmichael Low, who conducted field experiments on how mosquitoes transmitted malaria. As well as drawing mosquitoes, Terzi took part in an experiment whereby the three men spent many nights in a hut, screened against the mosquitoes. They did not contract malaria while those working out in the open in the same locality did, helping to confirm the theory that mosquitoes transmitted malaria.

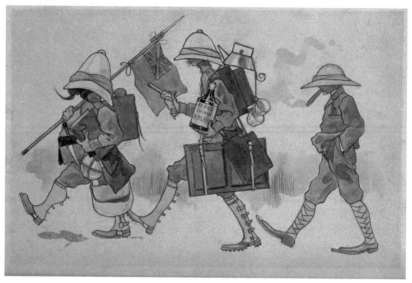

Figure 8.2 Three members of the Roman Campagna Malaria Commission carrying their gear (coloured pen drawing by A. Terzi, *c.* 1900)

Credit: Wellcome Library, London

What can we glean from this source about the responses to malaria in the early 1900s?

Feedback

The image is useful for portraying how the mosquito scientists viewed themselves. The turn of the century saw the introduction of practical applications of Ross's new theory. 'War' was waged against the mosquito, as exemplified by the use of 'Mosquito Brigades'. As Terzi actually joined some field researchers, he may have produced this image of them precisely because that was how they were acting. The cartoon is also representative of the development of the art of entomological illustration and the use of official artists.

What of the human populations? The clinical aspect of the disease in human populations and the challenge to reduce morbidity and mortality rested on a single pharmacological tool. For those humans who lived in malarious regions or who had contracted malaria, there was only one drug available – quinine. Made from cinchona bark, quinine had been brought to Europe in the seventeenth century as a cure for fever (Dobson, 1998). By the mid nineteenth century, quinine had been isolated from the cinchona bark and made available for prophylaxis and treatment. Understanding how quinine acted upon the parasites in humans was the major challenge. To this end, Robert Koch conducted quininization trials in Tanganyika, East Africa in the late nineteenth and early twentieth centuries to determine effect and dosage, perhaps the earliest field trials in sub-Saharan Africa, with inconclusive results. Quinine for prophylaxis and treatment was standard practice for the protection of soldiers throughout the colonial empires. Most soldiers had to be forced to ingest quinine given its bitter taste and the fear of getting blackwater fever, an almost always fatal disease tied to the use of quinine prophylaxis. In spite of these obstacles, there was huge success in reducing mortality. Soldiers were controlled populations and thus fairly stable in terms of proving the use and success of quinine. Would this strategy work to the same effect with civilian populations?

One of the most successful public health programmes to use quinine was conducted in Italy in the first decades of the twentieth century. In the late nineteenth century, the Italian government targeted the Roman Campagna, near the capital, Rome. It organized Ross-style mosquito brigades to pour oil on mosquito breeding sites to kill mosquito larvae and also engineered swamp drainage. Although malaria morbidity and mortality was reduced, significant malaria prevalence persisted. The government then turned to a two-pronged public health programme centred first on quinine distribution at subsidized cost to rural health centres. Then, following Celli's arguments, funds were allocated to create schools that would include malaria information in the general education curriculum. The combination of social development, environmental engineering and quinine prophylaxis was successful in significantly reducing malaria mortality but not morbidity. Sick workers remained an economic burden.

Following the First World War, the new Italian government under Mussolini introduced a programme termed 'bonification'. Land was reclaimed in the Roman Campagna and Pontine swamps to create new agricultural lands for poor Italian farmers and, strategically, to increase popular support for the Fascist government (Frost 1934; Packard, 2007). A second more extensive and heavily funded bonification programme included dam construction and water relocation. Thus reclaimed land was available for both settlement and agriculture. Towns were established with an infrastructure that included new roads, schools and hospitals resulting in population growth, economic development and, finally, significant reductions in malaria mortality. The plan rightfully was deemed successful in eliminating malaria from the targeted areas. The Italian Programme became the model for malaria control and eradication programmes elsewhere in Europe and the United States.

Exercise 8.4: Costs

During the 1930s the Italian Prime Minister Benito Mussolini spent 549 million lira to drain the Pontine swamps. This was the equivalent of US$400 million at 2005 prices (Packard, 2007, p. 131). Look at the graph below, which shows sources of funds spent on malaria control programmes worldwide, and then answer the questions that follow.

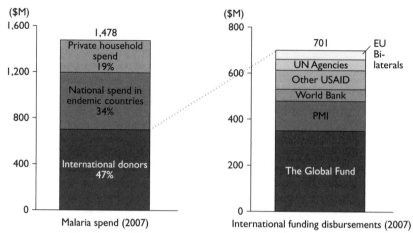

Figure 8.3 Current sources of funds spent on malaria

Source: Roll Back Malaria Partnership, The Global Malaria Action Plan, WHO 2008, URL: http://www.rollbackmalaria.org/gmap/1-4.html (accessed on 29 July 2011)

1   How do you think the amount spent in Italy in the 1930s compares with the expenditure on malaria control today?
2   Suggest some examples of the expenditure on malaria which the chart showing 'Malaria spend 2007' may represent. Are there also indirect costs of malaria not captured in this graph?

Feedback

1   This was a huge sum to spend by one individual country. Fascist Italy considered malaria a major economic hindrance and made its control a main priority. Today, countries may face a variety of health problems and malaria is not always considered the major health issue. HIV/AIDS, for example, in countries such as Botswana, is considered the priority. Figure 8.3 shows that a significant proportion of funds for malaria control in endemic regions comes from external sources. But malaria is a long-term issue perhaps requiring funding for 25 years or more.
2   Malaria has both direct and indirect costs. Direct personal expenditure might include insecticide-treated mosquito nets, doctors' fees, anti-malarial drugs, transport to health facilities, and support for the patient and family member during hospital stays. Public expenditures might include government expenditure on health facilities and health care infrastructure, vector control, education and research. Indirect costs include things such as loss of income and productivity due to sickness or death, and interruption of schooling as a result of illness.

From Italy to Africa

During the first thirty years of the twentieth century, Italian public health practitioners were not alone in incorporating environmental development strategies to address malaria. Similar strategies were adopted in the Panama Canal Zone, in the southern

United States, and in Russia in the wake of the malaria epidemic of 1922–1923. Epidemics that affected labouring populations triggered interest and research. Colonel S.P. James, the British Colonial Office advisor on malaria, visited East Africa following a serious epidemic in the late 1920s. Malaria had come to the Kenya Highlands, a high-altitude area thought to be too cold for malaria. When African labourers were struck more than once with the disease, economic considerations underwrote political action. James advocated social and economic development – screened windows on houses, drainage of water-lying areas, oiling of potential breeding sites. The timing was unfortunate as his recommendations, and the Colonial Office decision to invest in development, coincided with the onset of the Great Depression, which resulted in worldwide economic recession.

James' Report (James, 1929) had international ramifications. The League of Nations, established following the First World War, sponsored both a Malaria Commission and a Health Committee. James was the unacknowledged author of the Malaria Commission report to the Health Committee. The Malaria Commission followed the success of Mussolini's bonification programme with interest. The League and the Commission had no access to funding to sponsor programmes. In Kenya, neither the local settler-governed economy nor the Colonial Office could provide funding to carry out the Report's recommendations. James made a strong case for linking environmental and economic development to health policy for malaria. The Italian government proved this policy successful. Although military needs in the 1930s and 1940s stimulated the development of synthetic anti-malarial drugs, international interest in malaria and Africa had to await the 1950s reconstruction. Civilian populations were often unwilling participants. Malaria experiments were conducted in the Nazi concentration camps in Europe during the Second World War. Insecticides for typhus and louse control, reminiscent of earlier plague control measures, were used on civilian populations.

Strategies and tools II: 1940–1970

No other period in the last 150 years has seen the enthusiasm and optimism of the years after the Second World War. The League of Nations had been transformed into the United Nations and the Health Committee into the World Health Organization (WHO). Confident and well-funded, the WHO embarked upon an evidence-gathering project to address issues of health and disease at the global level to inform national and international policy. For malaria research, there emerged two exciting tools for malaria eradication. The first was chloroquine, a synthetic anti-malarial that could be used for prophylaxis, without the visible side-effects of earlier synthetic anti-malarials used during the Second World War such as atebrine. The second tool, dichlorodiphenyltrichloroethane (DDT), synthesized in 1874, was not designed for malaria control but for typhus. The Swiss scientist, P.H. Müller, awarded the Nobel Prize in Physiology or Medicine in 1948 for this research, transformed the pesticide into a powerful residual insecticide. Trials of DDT in Mexico and Kenya in the 1940s demonstrated its 'knock-off' effects – killing adult mosquitoes at contact and retaining potency on walls of huts for a minimum of three months in the field. The trials in East Africa gained popularity as DDT also killed bedbugs! The potential for reduction of Anopheles mosquitoes to below the level of significance for transmission had been proven – or proven to some.

In 1950, a WHO technical conference of malariologists was called to take place in Kampala, Uganda to discuss the challenges of establishing a Global Malaria Eradication Programme. The conference participants included, among other officials, local malaria field researchers, international malariologists and a representative from the Rockefeller Foundation, Paul Russell. Rockefeller-funded malaria eradication success, under the direction of Fred Soper, in Egypt and Sardinia drove the enthusiasm for taking DDT to a global eradication programme (Dobson, Malowany and Snow, 2000). George MacDonald, an eminent mathematical statistician at the London School of Hygiene and Tropical Medicine, worked out a mathematical formula linking mosquito reduction to reduced transmission. Using Macdonald's formula, the conference established definitions of degrees of endemicity to facilitate malaria control and comparative research (Dobson et al., 2000).

For the first time in an international forum, debates took place over the design of a malaria eradication programme. Field researchers in East Africa were wary of an eradication programme that did not take into account endemicity (i.e. the rate or intensity of transmission). Would an eradication programme in a high transmission area not interrupt the acquisition of immunity of African populations? If the programme failed, Africans would be increasingly vulnerable. The resolution was to go ahead with the global eradication programme. Sub-Saharan Africa, however, would be targeted for pre-eradication trials while full eradication programmes would be undertaken in India, Sardinia and other areas of malaria concern. In 1955, the WHO formally launched its first Global Malaria Eradication Program (GMEP) built on the two-pronged attack of DDT against the vector and chloroquine as human prophylaxis. Some of the participants were aware that resistance to DDT had been recently demonstrated and that its use on this scale had to be undertaken quickly and thoroughly. DDT was a tool with a limited lifespan.

Exercise 8.5

The final report of the 1950 Malaria Conference in Equatorial Africa, held in Kampala, 'recommends to governments responsible for the administration of African territories that malaria should be controlled by modern methods as soon as feasible, whatever the original degree of endemicity, and without awaiting the outcome of further experiments' (WHO, 1951).

Consider the quotations below and then answer the questions that follow.

Quotation 1

'A major control scheme in a hyperendemic area of Africa might be followed by malaria of a different character, and of much more serious import, than that to which we are accustomed, if control measures slackened.'

D.B. Wilson, clinician and malariologist (Wilson, Garnham and Swellengrebel, 1950, p. 694)

Quotation 2

'Go ahead by all means but be sure that you can bring your work to a successful end.'
D.B. Wilson, P.C.C. Garnham and N.H. Swellengrebel (WHO Afr/Mal/Conf/25.62)

Quotation 3

'In 1950, the first African malaria conference of WHO was held in Kampala, principally to discuss the policy of malaria eradication by spraying dwellings with DDT ... Furious debates arose ... I shall never forget how Leonard (Bruce-Chwatt) poured oil on troubled waters, by folding his hands and quietly saying "Let us spray".

P.C.C. Garnham, parasitologist (Garnham, 1989, p. 68)

Quotation 4

'Hyperendemic malaria was grossly damaging to all concerned and, therefore, in urgent need of control. Immunity of the African, he argued, was purchased at too great a cost in mortality and morbidity, adding: "there is a grave responsibility involved in withholding control measures – in short – we have the devices of control now, so why don't we use them?"'

George McDonald (WHO Registry files, WHO.2. DC. Mal. 20. Africa Reports, no author)

1 What concerns were being raised about the potential malaria programmes?
2 Comment on the value of these quotations as historical sources.

Feedback

1 The quotations highlight the debate behind the recommendation of the final report. Quotations 1 and 2 highlight concerns of the long-term effect of control policies. In this case the fear was that control policies would not be completed or successful, potentially leaving areas worse off than prior to the campaign. A critical debate that had emerged had been the issue of 'natural immunity' to malaria and the link between immunity and endemicity. Concerns included that intervention in areas of high malaria transmission might lead to a loss of naturally acquired immunity, which could give rise to a resurgence of malaria, if control strategies were not sustained. Quotations 3 and 4 highlight the pressure to act now. Tools such as DDT had become available to combat malaria and some scientists urged that it was unethical to withhold such tools.
2 The use of so-called 'grey literature' (non-commercially published material such as reports) and sources including diaries, transcripts and interviews, can provide a valuable additional resource to published reports. Caution, however, is also needed when cross-referencing sources taking into account issues such as memory loss and bias.

The GMEP goal was malaria eradication – that is, the reduction of infected mosquitoes, transmission of the parasite, and ultimately eradication of the disease in the human population. Vector control measures, oiling and water breeding site inspection, so important in the early twentieth century, were not part of the funded programme. Delivery was vertical – targeting Anopheles mosquitoes in multiple areas of endemicity. The GMEP was not incorporated into government health delivery programmes or practice. Funding and technical assistance was provided through the WHO and a second United Nations specialized agency, UNICEF. The budget for DDT was based on a twice-yearly spraying. For island areas, this was sufficient to reduce adult-biting mosquitoes and interrupt transmission to reduce both morbidity and mortality. For other more rural areas, Uganda or Nigeria, for example, field malariologists reported that they needed to spray every three months. And they did, thus emptying the insecticide supplies earlier than budgeted. When requests were sent for renewed insecticides, the budget had been spent. By 1969, fourteen years after the launch of the programme, it was quietly withdrawn. Research reported the development of chloroquine resistance and the cost of finding alternative anti-malarials was more than the WHO or UNICEF could fund. In the United States, a new environmental movement had grown around the writings of Rachel Carson and her 1962 publication, *Silent Spring*, challenging the use of DDT as a poison with possible carcinogenic long-term effects. There would be no renewal of funding from the United States for the Global Programme.

The Global Malaria Eradication Programme concluded with mixed results. It was successful in economically developed states (Italy, Netherlands, Spain, Portugal, for example) or on islands (Grenada, Puerto Rico, Cuba), where the possibility of reducing the total number of mosquitoes was an achievable goal. As sub-Saharan Africa was not part of the Programme, the area with the greatest disease burden remained a challenge. During the years of the GMEP, partly due to the 'magic bullet' optimism attached to the tool, DDT, entomological research diminished in funding and practice. Indeed, the Programme is said to have 'eradicated malariologists'. Governments, particularly in Africa, that previously had allocated funds for vector control virtually eliminated these costs from their budget. This tactic removed the costs but not the problem. Such was the unbridled optimism or certainty of success with DDT and chloroquine that malaria research had practically come to a standstill.

For the two decades after the conclusion of the GMEP, malaria disappeared from the global health agenda. New African states had other priorities. Frequent and problematic economic fluctuations, oil crises and government changes all contributed to keeping malaria in the background. Better scientific laboratory tools and the political will of scientific researchers, from the South and North, brought the challenge of malaria back to the scientific research and health policy tables in the 1990s.

Strategies and tools III: 1990s to present

Two scientific meetings, in Amsterdam in 1992 and Dakar in 1996, provided the impetus to bring malaria control and eradication to the WHO for consideration and action. Health ministers joined scientists from the north and south to work out a 'Global Strategy for Malaria Control'. Under the leadership of Dr. Gro Harlem Brundtland, the WHO launched the Roll Back Malaria (RBM) programme in 1998 to provide the framework for this strategy and to deliver interventions to achieve the goal of malaria eradication. The RBM was designed as a horizontal programme, building on the WHO's commitment to primary health care. The goal was thought to be achievable: reducing malaria mortality by 50 per cent by 2010. This time, Africa was included. Taking lessons from the successful smallpox eradication programme, RBM sought to include education and training of health workers, paying particular attention to training within existing state health delivery infrastructures. Pharmaceutical companies demonstrated willingness to meet RBM goals through research funding for vaccines and, innovatively, for combination therapies for malaria prophylaxis. The scientific world was well aware that resistance to existing anti-malarials was growing, with chloroquine practically ineffective in many parts of the malarious world.

Two new innovations on old tools became part of RBM strategies. Although the programme set specific targets for children under five, the WHO realized that the target populations for prevention would have to include families, communities and villages. The RBM was designed to be a global public health intervention programme with local and regional variations or adaptations. With regard to health policy, governments were encouraged to develop a malaria programme that addressed prevention, control and treatment. National policies for malaria chemoprophylaxis and treatment were encouraged (i.e. to specify which drugs would be reserved for first and second line treatment and which drugs made available for prophylaxis). Resistance to known anti-malarials had been documented. Innovative combination drugs and sound malaria policies would lengthen the life and use of available anti-malarials. Termed combination therapies, these new approaches would include a rediscovered anti-malarial plant, *Artemisia annua*, indigenous to China and easily adaptable to other soils and climates, especially to the agricultural areas of sub-Saharan Africa. In the long term, African countries would be able to produce their own pharmacological therapies (Duffy and Mutabingwa, 2006).

The second innovation added a brilliant twist to an ancient protective tool, the bed net. Whereas bed nets had prevented mosquitoes from biting humans sleeping under them, the reinvented bed nets would be dipped in pyrethrum, a natural insecticide, adding mosquito control to human protection while sleeping under the net. Insecticide treated nets (ITNs), locally manufactured and distributed, were an affordable, portable and sustainable tool. However, as with every other malaria control innovation, even the ITNs courted controversy. It was an old question – raised by S.P. James in the 1930s, in 1950 in Kampala and in the 1990s – concerning endemicity, transmission rates, the acquisition or loss of immunity. Could an intervention tool be used across areas of varying endemicity/transmission? (Dobson et al., 2000). The most exciting results came from trials conducted in The Gambia, which showed that the use of ITNs reduced all-cause child mortality (ages 1–4) by 60 per cent. Trial results also showed a reduction in malaria-caused mortally in children ages 0–3 by 17 per cent, ages 1–4 by 33 per cent and ages 1–9 by 14 per cent (Greenwood, 1993).

Such results encouraged WHO to back the widespread application of ITNs without regard to endemicity. Once more it appeared that any concern with local variations in endemicity and disease transmission had been overshadowed by the hope of offering a single and cost-effective measure of control across wide areas.

Exercise 8.6

Study the following quotation from Bill Gates' keynote address to the Malaria Forum in 2007, and then answer the questions that follow.

'What is the most repeated failure in all of global health? It could well be the commitment to eradicate malaria. So why would anyone want to follow a long line of failures by becoming the umpteenth person to declare the goal of eradicating malaria? There is one reason. We should declare the goal of eradicating malaria because we can eradicate malaria. Today, I want to make the case that we have a real chance to build the partnerships, generate the political will and develop the scientific breakthroughs we need to end this disease.'

1 What does this source indicate about attitudes to malaria and the interests involved?
2 What problems might be faced by these new attempts at eradication?

Feedback

1 The quotation reflects the re-invigoration of attempts to control malaria that developed in the 1990s. The source highlights the role of private interests in re-shaping the malaria field, in this instance Gates – the wealthy philanthropist who poured money into the arena. After 2007 the concept of malaria eradication and elimination emerged on the global health agenda. The optimism around malaria control is also related to the emergence of new anti-malarial therapeutics such as *Artemisia annua* and its derivative Artemisinin, which have provided an additional tool to combat malaria, and the new insecticide impregnated bed nets provide community-based, affordable prevention. As with DDT and chloroquine, these tools re-established hope that malaria control was possible.

2 Problems that may prevent eradication include poverty, resistance to insecticides and drugs, population movements, war, lack of community involvement, poor statistics and surveillance, the complexity of the parasite and of very high transmission rates particularly in sub-Saharan Africa. Some malariologists have raised concerns and suggest this approach of eradication is too ambitious; elimination would be a more appropriate end goal.

In 2005, the RBM Partnership brought together international donors and foundations to work with the WHO. This dynamic collaboration has provided the basis for monitoring and evaluating RBM targets and delivery, while also providing opportunities and funds to design and facilitate the implementation of new public health interventions. The delivery of these interventions, and the creation of public health policies, rests with the governments of those countries affected by malaria. On the ground or in the field, economic uncertainties, fluctuating political will and constrained health budgets militate against timely success. In spite of the difficulties, the programme has achieved unprecedented success in establishing malaria as a global health challenge. The RBM Partnership, Millennium Development Goals, Global Fund to Fight AIDS, TB and Malaria, and the Gates-funded Global Health Group have consolidated funding, aims, strategies and tools. They have also provided encouragement to pharmaceutical companies to engage in malaria research and malaria vaccine trials. Fighting malaria – malaria control, eradication and elimination – has been included within larger global health goals that include better evidence, evidence-based policy and international agreements incorporating a public health and health systems perspective.

The use of history or history and policy

What have we learned from the past? Contemporary interventions address the complexity of transmission, endemicity and infection in addition to challenges of access, infrastructure and health care-disease prevention capability and delivery. Malaria research in the laboratory and in the field, together with the design and practice of interventions, maintains a multi-level focus on malaria that includes the contexts in which people, parasites and mosquitoes live and interact. The 'magic bullet' approach to malaria is in the past. The remaining question and challenge is to select the malaria programme that best suits the epidemiological, political and economic realities to keep the long-term goal of sustainability at the forefront.

Summary

We return to the original set of puzzle pieces: human populations, vectors and parasites. We place these pieces within the complex environments that include communities and cities, countries and regions to consider how to address the challenge of malaria control, eradication or management to elimination. We recognize that there are multiple possible responses to reflect the complexity of the puzzle but we want to implement the best responses – best practice based on best evidence (*The Lancet, Malaria Elimination Series*, 2010). Combination therapeutics, insecticide treated nets and rapid testing for malaria diagnostics have contributed to the tool kit. We need to continue to refine and improve these developments, including the search for a vaccine. The answers remain as complex as malaria itself.

References and further reading

Alonso PL, Lindsay SW, Armstrong Schellenberg JRM, Keita K, Gomez P, Shenton FC, Hill AG, David PH, Fegan G, Cham K and Greenwood BM (1993) A malaria control trial using insecticide-treated bed nets and targeted chemoprophylaxis in a rural area of The Gambia, West Africa. 6. The impact of the interventions on mortality and morbidity from malaria, *Transactions of the Royal Society of Tropical Medicine and Hygiene*, 87(suppl. 2): 37–44.

Bynum WF (1999) Ronald Ross and the malaria–mosquito cycle, *Parassitologia*, 41(1–3): 49–52.

Carson R (1962) *Silent Spring*. New York: Houghton Mifflin.

Coluzzi M and Bradley D (eds) (1999) The Malaria Challenge after one hundred years of malariology. Papers from the Malariology Centenary Conference, Accademia Nazionale dei Lincei, Roma, 16–19 November 1998, *Parassitologia*, 41(1–3).

Dobson MJ (1998) Bitter-sweet solutions for malaria: Exploring natural remedies from the past, *Parassitologia*, 40(1–2): 69–81.

Dobson MJ (1999) The Malariology Centenary, *Parassitologia*, 41(1–3): 31–2.

Dobson MJ, Malowany M and Snow RW (2000) Malaria control in East Africa: The Kampala Conference and the Pare-Taveta Scheme: A meeting of common and high ground, *Parassitologia*, 42(1–2): 149–66.

Duffy PE and Mutabingwa TK (2006) Artemisinin combination therapies, *Lancet*, 367(9528): 2037–9.

Fantini B (1999) The concept of specificity and the Italian contribution to the discovery of the malaria transmission cycle, *Parassitologia*, 41(3): 39–47.

Gallup JL and Sachs JD (2001) The economic burden of malaria, *American Journal of Tropical Medicine and Hygiene*, 64: 85–96.

Garnham PCC (supervising director) (1946) *DDT Versus Malaria: A Successful Experiment in Malaria Control by the Kenya Medical Department*. Film produced by the Kenya Medical Department, Electronic Source. London: Wellcome Trust Film Library.

Garnham PCC (1989) Professor L.J. Bruce-Chwatt's 80th birthday, *Journal of Tropical Medicine and Hygiene*, 92: 67–70.

Goodman CA, Coleman PG and Mills AJ (1999) Cost-effectiveness of malaria control in sub-Saharan Africa, *Lancet*, 354(9176): 378–85.

Greenwood BM (1993) Summary and conclusions: A malaria control trial using insecticide-treated bed nets and targeted chemoprophylaxis in a rural area of The Gambia, West Africa, *Transactions of the Royal Society of Tropical Medicine and Hygiene*, 87(suppl. 2): 59–60.

Hackett LW (1937) *Malaria in Europe: An Ecological Study*. London: Oxford University Press.

James SP (1929) *Report on a Visit to Kenya and Uganda to Advise on Anti-malarial Measures*. London: Crown Agents for the Colonies.

Litsios S (1996) *The Tomorrow of Malaria*. Wellington, NZ: Pacific Press.

Manson P (1898) Surgeon-Major Ronald Ross's recent investigations on the mosquito-malaria theory, *British Medical Journal*, 1: 1575–7.

Packard R (1998) No other logical choice: Malaria eradication and the politics of international health, *Parassitologia*, 40: 217–30.

Packard R (2007) *The Making of a Tropical Disease: A Short History of Malaria*. Baltimore, MD: The Johns Hopkins University Press.

Powers H (1997) Drug resistant malaria: A global problem and the Thai response, in Cunningham A (ed) *Western Medicine as Contested Knowledge* (pp. 262–8). Manchester: Manchester University Press.

Snow RW, Okiro EA, Gething PW, Atun R and Hay SI (2010) Equity and adequacy of international donor assistance for global malaria control: An analysis of populations at risk and external funding commitments, *Lancet*, 376(9750): 1368–70.

Snowden F (2006) *The Conquest of Malaria in Italy, 1900–1962*. New Haven, CT: Yale University Press.

Steketee R and Campbell C (2010) Impact of national malaria control scale-up programmes in Africa: Magnitude and attribution of effects, *Malaria Journal*, 9: 299.

Webb JLA, Jr. (2009) *Humanity's Burden: A Global History of Malaria*. Cambridge: Cambridge University Press.

Willcox M, Bodeker G and Rasaoanaivo P (eds) (2004) *Traditional Medicinal Plants and Malaria*. Boca Raton, FL: CRC Press.

Wilson DB, Garnham PCC and Swellengrebel NH (1950) A review of hyperendemic malaria, *Tropical Diseases Bulletin*, 47: 677–98.

World Health Organization (1951) Report of the Malaria Conference in Equatorial Africa, *WHO Technical Report Series*, 38: 1–72. Geneva: WHO.

Dedicated Journals or Special Issues:

Malaria Journal

American Journal of Tropical Medicine and Hygiene (2007) Volume 77, No. 6 (supplement), Defining and Defeating the Intolerable Burden of Malaria III.

The Lancet. Malaria Elimination Series, 2010. Access: www.ploscollections.org/malERA2011

SECTION 3

Twentieth century

Health systems and welfare states in the West, 1880s–1960s

9

Martin Gorsky

Overview

In this chapter, we move away from specific case studies and once again pick up the thread of the development of public health in the West. The evolution of public health can be seen in conjunction with the development of health systems and the welfare state. This chapter provides an introduction to the history of twentieth century health systems in the advanced industrial nations. The central theme is the growing role of the state in either organizing or directly providing health services, and in facilitating access to them for its citizens. The narrative is bookended by two milestones: 1883, when Bismarck established national health insurance in Germany, and 1965 when the USA passed the Medicare and Medicaid legislation. After a brief survey of health services in the nineteenth century, we provide a factual account of key legislative developments in three case-study countries: Germany exemplifies social insurance arrangements, Britain the single-payer 'national health service' (NHS) system, and the USA a mixed system with greater reliance on private insurance and individualism. We then discuss leading theoretical approaches to explaining these developments.

Learning objectives

After working through this chapter, you will be able to:

- recognize some key policy developments in the field of health service provision and financing in selected Western nations between the late nineteenth and early twentieth centuries
- identify and synthesize historical explanations for these developments
- critically analyse primary and secondary sources related to health system histories

Key terms

Single-payer system Description of systems where the funding of health services is organized in a single 'pool' that covers the whole population, and in which financing may be on an insurance basis or through direct taxation. This contrasts

> with the 'third-party payer' systems of social insurance, where multiple insurance funds collect and pay for health services on behalf of citizen and state.
>
> **Social insurance** State-mandated membership of a health insurance fund (whether private, mutual or public), typically managed through payroll deduction.

Introduction

In Chapter 3, we saw how economic modernization in the nineteenth century was increasingly accompanied by state intervention in various aspects of public health. We now explore the more extensive role played by governments in the twentieth century in establishing health systems. Since the beginning, the medical encounter between doctor and patient had typically been a commercial transaction, with access and quality determined by market power. Modern health systems sought to regulate those transactions so that an ever-wider pool of the population was eligible for care, and the delivery of health services was no longer market-driven. As in Chapters 2 and 3, this will be explored through national case studies. Germany illustrates the 'Bismarck system', named after the German Chancellor who introduced the world's first national health insurance (NHI) programme. Britain, with its comprehensive, universal, free and tax-funded service exemplifies the so-called 'Beveridge system' (a misattribution, as the economist and social reformer William Beveridge played little part in founding the NHS). The United States meanwhile is often seen as an outlier, because it was much slower in legislating for universal coverage, and preferred to build provision through the private and non-profit sectors. This chapter aims first to show what happened, and then to look at explanations for why.

The development of health systems

The first milestone came in 1883, shortly after German Unification, when Chancellor Otto von Bismarck successfully introduced the *Gesetz betreffend die Krankenversicherung der Arbeiter* (Law concerning the Health Insurance of the Worker). This made it compulsory for manual labourers to take out health insurance, with costs split between employers and employees, to cover them for sickness benefit and medical care when ill.

Exercise 9.1 The motives of German policy-makers

Read the extract below from the Imperial Message to the Reichstag (Parliament), delivered on 17 November 1881 by Kaiser (King) Wilhelm II, but representing Bismarck's ideas. Then answer the question that follows.

> 'Already in February of this year we expressed our conviction that the curing of social ills cannot be achieved solely through the repression of social-democratic [i.e. socialist] excesses but requires also positive promotion of the workers' well-being. We hold it to be our imperial duty to lay this responsibility anew before the

Reichstag. We should be able to look back on all the successes which God has so evidently granted to our government with all the more satisfaction if we are able to know in our hearts that we could leave behind to the fatherland new and permanent bastions of internal peace and content and to provide those who need help with greater security and a larger measure of the assistance to which they are entitled ...

In this sense the draft law on insurance of workers against industrial accidents put forward at the last session by the confederated governments will be revised in the light of the discussions in the Reichstag, in order to prepare a new version thereof. It will be supplemented by a draft proposal for a similar organisation on insurance schemes against occupational diseases. Furthermore, those who are incapacitated for work due to old age and disability also have a claim on the community for a higher level of state-provided assistance than has so far been their lot.

Finding the right ways and means to provide such assistance is a difficult task, but also one of the noblest that can be undertaken by any community that rests on the ethical foundations of a nation with a Christian way of life.'

(Bauriedl, 1981, p. 403)

• For what reasons did Bismarck believe social protection for the worker was necessary?

Feedback

Three main issues stand out. First, Bismarck was worried about social conflict arising from the demands of the organized working class (the 'social democrats'). In addition to suppressing left-wing troublemakers, he wanted to give concessions that would damp down rebellion and satisfy the workers' aspirations (note the reference to 'entitlement'). Second, the focus of legislation would be the industrial worker, not the population at large, suggesting a concern with economic efficiency. Third, the ethical justification was Christian morality.

However, we cannot automatically assume that the Message gives a direct insight into Bismarck's motives. The speech is designed to win over the support of the Reichstag, and had to be acceptable to the Kaiser. In fact, recent work on Bismarck's private papers has revealed that it was the second of these motives that was crucial, and the reference to the threat of socialism was intended mainly to win political support for the measures.

In time, this German innovation would become the basis of universal health coverage in many nations, and inspire the programmes of 'community-based health insurance' championed by development economists today. However, both publicly funded health care and the idea of group health insurance have a history long predating Bismarck.

Before Bismarck

The principle of workers clubbing together to save money for funeral costs or times of ill-health goes back more than three hundred years. Organizational structures originated with the trade guilds, formal associations of skilled workers, and their successors, the journeymen's clubs that were the antecedents of modern trade unions. In Britain, they developed beyond specific industries as 'friendly societies': grassroots 'self-help' associations of workers from different backgrounds. In Prussia, the largest of the German states prior to the country's unification, the funds (*Hilfskassen*) were based in the community and workplace. America, too, had a rich culture of fraternities, although these were more geared to sociability than welfare; however, work-based 'industrial assurance' sick funds were common in urbanized regions. Therefore, it was civil society and organized labour that pioneered health insurance, although they did not extend coverage universally, and favoured male industrial workers in stable employment.

Public provision of hospitals also dates at least to the late seventeenth century, with the building of the English workhouses and early American almshouses. These were institutions for the confinement of the poor, which, in practice, also provided hospital care. The eighteenth century saw the first foundations of acute care and teaching hospitals funded by philanthropy, many of which have survived to the present. The result was that, particularly in the United States and Britain, a two-tier system developed, with a stigmatized and badly funded poor law sector offering long-term care to impoverished older people and psychiatric patients, and a more prestigious and scientifically oriented voluntary sector of hospitals catering to the 'respectable' poor. This was not the model everywhere: in Scandinavia local government tended to fund general hospitals for all, while in Germany university and municipal hospitals were publicly supported.

However, until the end of the nineteenth century therapies were fairly limited, with nursing, bed rest and the palliative use of opiates to the fore. Then the hospital began to transform itself. Safe anaesthesia, Joseph Lister's development of antisepsis and new blood transfusion technology opened up vistas of possibility for surgery, which had hitherto been confined to techniques such as cutting for gallstones. The X-ray machine, and from the 1930s radiotherapy for cancer patients, similarly confirmed the hospital's new identity as centre of scientific technology. The 'bacteriological revolution' and subsequent microbiological discoveries of Pasteur and Koch were followed in the 1930s by the sulphonamides (drugs that inhibit bacterial reproduction) and in the 1940s by antibiotics. Thus hospital medicine changed from charitable relief for the poor into something desired by all social classes, and this raised new questions for governments about how to ensure access and provision.

Germany

Germany developed its health system through the gradual expansion of social insurance. Hospitals were organized mostly in the public and non-profit sectors, with some private, while physicians were independent providers, either employed by hospitals or contracting with sick funds on the basis of fee for service.

- 1883: Start of National Health Insurance (NHI) – maternity care, sick and death pay, time-limited in- and out-patient care, free drugs.
- 1900: Sick fund doctors formed *Hartmannbund*, a trade union to defend pay and conditions.
- 1911–1914: NHI extended to civil servants, transport, office and agricultural workers; population coverage increased from 20 per cent to 30 per cent, in *c.* 22,000 separate *Krankenkassen* (sick funds).
- 1913: Berlin Treaty. An agreement between state and doctors established committee structure to resolve employment disputes with funds.
- 1914: Implementation of *Reichsversicherungsordnung* (Imperial Insurance Code), which regulates NHI.

- 1918: Coverage for unemployed; new obstetric and midwifery benefits.
- 1930: Full coverage for dependants.
- 1933–1945: Third Reich – workers lost majorities on fund committees, Jewish doctors persecuted.
- 1941: Coverage for pensioners.
- 1966: Coverage for farmers and salespersons.
- 1972–1975: Inclusion of self-employed and dependants, students; further consolidation means now only c. 1600 funds covering c. 90 per cent of population; those on high incomes excluded – they are insured privately.

Britain

Britain adopted a limited version of the Bismarck model, excluding hospital benefits to avoid undermining voluntary sector philanthropy. In the inter-war period, dissatisfaction grew about gaps in coverage and the inefficiencies of multiple providers. During the Second World War, planning for reform accelerated. This led to the NHS Acts, sometimes characterized as a 'big-bang' reform because they fundamentally changed arrangements for financing and provision.

- 1906–1911: Liberal welfare reforms – school meals, school medical service, old age pensions.
- 1911: National Health Insurance Act. Friendly societies became agents of NHI. They provided sickness benefit and primary care, but no hospital treatment and costs were split between employee, employer and government.
- 1920s: Rise of independent voluntary sector hospital contributory schemes for working class.
- 1929: Local Government Act. Poor law administration dismantled; municipal and county councils took over poor law infirmaries with many run as general hospitals; stigma was reduced and quality improved.
- 1942: Beveridge Report. Published in wartime with a blueprint for a universalist welfare state to tackle the 'five giant evils' of unemployment, poor education and housing, ill-health and poverty. Beveridge's 'Assumption B' was that a comprehensive health service would be created, but no concrete proposals were made.
- 1944: NHS White Paper. Document issued by coalition government containing reform proposals. Legislation stalled due to opposition from British Medical Association and voluntary hospital leaders.
- 1945: Labour Party unexpectedly won large parliamentary majority.
- 1946–1947: NHS Acts carried through Parliament by Labour Minister of Health, Aneurin Bevan. Hospitals taken into national ownership; population coverage universal; private medicine allowed but most physicians contract to state scheme; funding by direct taxation.
- 1948: NHS starts.

United States

Americans looked at the European example but did not adopt it, with the result that coverage grew either through non-profit insurance or through employment based organizations. Mid-century attempts to introduce NHI also failed, although in the 1960s a more limited scheme for the elderly and the poor was introduced.

- 1910s: American Association for Labor Legislation lobbied for health insurance law modelled on Germany. Ohio, Pennsylvania, Illinois and New York state legislatures considered but rejected.
- 1917: California referendum on health insurance proposal defeated by 358,000 to 133,000.
- 1930s–1940s: Growth of voluntary sector Blue Cross and Blue Shield schemes to provide hospital and health care insurance. By 1945, 15.7 million enrolled in Blue Cross.
- 1935: New Deal: Social Security Bill. President Roosevelt decided not to include NHI alongside old age pensions and unemployment insurance.
- 1938: Industrialist Henry Kaiser established health fund for workers building the Grand Coulee Dam (the forerunner of Kaiser Permanente and later Health Maintenance Organizations).
- 1939, 1943, 1945, 1949: NHI proposed in Wagner, Murray, Dingell bills and Truman Plan, but rejected.
- 1945: Hill Burton Act. Public financing for private hospital building in under-supplied areas.
- 1965: Medical Care and Social Security Act. Established Medicare to cover over-65s and Medicaid to provide federal/state funding for welfare recipients and 'medically indigent'.

Explaining change: Health systems in welfare states

As the timelines above hint, the arrival of modern health systems was part of a larger process of the coming of welfare states in the West. What do we mean by a 'welfare state'? The historian Asa Briggs described it as follows:

A welfare state is a state in which organized power is deliberately used to modify the play of market forces in at least three directions – first, guaranteeing individuals a minimum income irrespective of the market value of their work or their property; second, by narrowing the extent of insecurity by enabling individuals to meet certain 'social contingencies' (for example, sickness, old age and unemployment) which lead otherwise to individual and family crises; and third, ensuring that all citizens, without distinction of status or class are offered the best standards available in relation to a certain agreed range of social services.

(Briggs, 1961, p. 228)

Thus in practice we are talking about the arrival of publicly funded programmes to provide pensions, social security payments, housing, education and of course health services. This has been a major historical transformation, involving a considerable transfer of resources from rich to poor, and it has generated a great deal of theorizing about why!

Economic modernization

As you saw in Chapter 3, the growth of state intervention can be understood in the broadest terms as part of the coming of urban, industrial society. In predominantly agrarian economies with small, stable populations, it was possible for social welfare to be left to the family and community, supplemented by religious charity and the obligation of landowners to provide for their labourers. With industrialization and growing, mobile populations, those ties and supports were removed. Now the workers were on their own, in labour contracts with employers whose only duty was to pay a money wage and where there was just the minimal safety net of philanthropy or poor law for those who failed. Yet as urbanization intensified and the problems of poverty and sickness grew more overt, so it became clear that market mechanisms alone were insufficient to deliver the social goods people needed. Welfare states were the response to this failure. In Karl Polanyi's words, society underwent a 'change to social and national protectionism ... due to the manifestation of the weaknesses and perils inherent in a self-regulating market system' (Polanyi, 2001, p. 152).

This general explanation would probably be acceptable to all but the most ardent free-marketeers, but although it gives an overarching context it does not take us very far. It implies the changes were simply inevitable, and it tells us nothing about why they happened when they did, or why different countries took different paths.

Marxist theory: Legitimation

One possible answer arises from the Marxist view that historical change in industrial society is driven by class conflict. The argument is that the huge inequalities between capitalists and labourers generated growing tensions and ultimately calls for social transformation, as employees sought a just share of the surplus wealth created by mechanization. Workers mobilized and agitated by forming trade unions, and ultimately political parties to represent their interests – in Germany the Social Democrats and in Britain the Labour Party. Faced with this, the ruling class had to devise policies that would defuse a potentially revolutionary situation. The health systems of welfare states were part of the answer. They were a concession of social benefits, which legitimized the inequitable structures of capitalism.

What is the evidence for this? We have already seen that Bismarck's Imperial Message talked frankly about NHI as a device for 'curing' social stresses, and other examples can be found. The theory is also useful for explaining why America did *not* adopt NHI at the same time as its European peers. In the United States, no genuinely left-wing party ever gained wide support, and militant organized labour was less threatening: trade unions were fractured by race and ethnicity, and dissatisfied workers could always 'go West' in search of opportunity. So here there was no such need for a legitimation strategy.

Exercise 9.2 The New Liberal programme in Britain

The extract below comes from a document often considered the first manifesto for the 'New' Liberalism. It was the Liberal Party that initiated Britain's welfare state in the early twentieth century with measures like school meals, old age pensions and NHI. The extract comes from a chapter discussing the importance of housing reform to health. Once you have read it, answer the question below.

'The evil effects of overcrowding upon the poorer classes of our large towns is now generally recognised, but it is not so widely understood that it is to the interest of all in the community to do away with these evils. Self-interest enforces the dictates of humanity. For under such conditions of life the workman, even if looked upon merely as an instrument to produce wealth, is not nearly so valuable to the community as he might be. The result of the improvements undertaken in Paris under Napoleon has been to reduce the mortality by one-half. But medical statistics show that for every person who dies in this way, six persons are ill, and the consequent loss to the community of wealth-producing power is enormous. The interests of one class cannot be separated from those of another ... The contagion of some disorders, influenza, for instance, is remarkable for its "amazing diffusibility", while that of others, such as scarlet fever, "remain dormant for months in articles of clothing". Now it must be borne in mind that the milk, the food, the linen used in the better classes pass through the hands of those who live in courts and alleys, and whose conditions of lives, although concealed, have the most serious influence upon the lives and health of those whose circumstances appear to place them above all danger, and who may live at a great distance from the source of contagion.

While re-housing may be looked upon as an insurance paid by the better class against disease, it may also be regarded as an insurance paid by the rich against revolution. It is useless to increase wages and to lessen the hours of toil so long as the workman is compelled to live in the pest-houses we have described; nay, it is almost worse than useless, inasmuch as the extra wage and increased leisure operate as incentives to drunkenness and vice. It is to the interest of all in the community that the workman should become a better instrument of production, that his dwelling should not be a hotbed of disease, that his degradation and misery should not be a constant source of danger to the State. The warning of Danton must be heeded, "If you suffer the poor to grow up as animals they may chance to become wild beasts and rend you".'

(Liberal Federation, 1885, pp. 78–80)

• To what extent do the arguments presented here support the 'legitimation' thesis?

Feedback

The source comes from 1885, so cannot be treated as direct evidence about the 1906–1911 welfare legislation. However, it does date from the same period as Bismarck's initiatives so could be used as a more general indicator of why public intervention in health was desirable in the proto-welfare state era.

The second paragraph apparently provides unequivocal vindication of the legitimation thesis, with the argument that social reform is 'insurance ... against revolution' (note how the interests of the 'rich' are treated as synonymous with those of the 'State'). There is also acknowledgement that better pay alone is insufficient to solve the problem of health and housing: the state must act where the market has failed.

However, the context suggests that legitimation was *not* the overriding interest of politicians. Indeed, the 'self-interest' of the state had two other elements. First, there was the concern for productivity, with reference to France's experience of housing reform successfully reducing morbidity. Second, a more direct threat to the rich than revolution came from infectious diseases, which might be transmitted from the poor through service industries like laundries or food preparation.

Legitimation theory may be useful for explaining some welfare state development. However, apart from the problem of demonstrating that it was the single most important motive, one big question remains. Could social peace not have been purchased at a rather cheaper cost to the rich than through the extensive universal systems that were created?

Marxist theory: Productivism

Some Marxist historians put greater emphasis on welfare states as a support for economic productivity, which we have just seen was a concern of both Bismarck and the New Liberals. The key argument is that state intervention was not inspired by human rights or compassion for others. Instead, it was needed by industrialists to guarantee the smooth running of capitalist economies. Health systems ensured that 'human capital' was well maintained and sickness would not reduce industrial output. Similarly, public education programmes would produce a well-educated workforce, while pensions and social security meant that the labour market could be regulated and demand for goods maintained during economic downturns.

Exercise 9.3 The early campaign for American social insurance

The extract below comes from the United States during the American Association for Labor Legislation's unsuccessful campaign, and represents the case made to the New Jersey legislature for introducing social health insurance. Once you have read the extract, answer the questions below.

> '*Extent of sickness in New Jersey.* Reliable indications … are found in the Community Sickness Survey of Trenton. According to their findings 3.1 per cent of all persons 15 years old and over were sick, and 2.4 per cent of all persons were so sick that they were unable to work. Estimates based on these figures indicate that in the course of a year sickness causes an annual loss of 7.2 working days to persons 15 years of age and that there are at all times 43,000 persons of 15 years and over who are so sick as to be unable to work. [I]n a single year among 1,500 New Jersey glass blowers there were 300 cases of sickness causing a loss of 10,000 working days …
>
> *The serious import of extensive sickness.* The draft [compulsory military service], with its alarming percentage of rejections because of physical deficiency, has aroused the country and driven home the fact that widely prevalent sickness is of national concern. An Official Bulletin recently issued by the Government states that out of approximately 1,300,000 volunteers for the Army and Navy since war was declared, but 448,859 were physically qualified, the rejection rate being 66 per cent …
>
> *Sickness and industry.* Although sickness is a problem for the community as a whole, it has an important industrial aspect. There appears to be a direct correlation between sickness and industrial conditions, as well as between sickness and wages. The potteries, smelters, tanneries, textile and hatting trades of New Jersey tell a tale of lead poisoning, mercury poisoning, and well known occupational diseases, but also of consumption, pneumonia and kindred ailments induced by work in dust or in humid atmosphere …'
>
> Source: New Jersey Commission (1917) *Report on
> Health Insurance by the New Jersey Commission*

1 What arguments are advanced about the problems of sickness?
2 What can the source tell us about productivist assumptions?

Feedback

1 In a more sophisticated echo of the Chadwick Report (Chapter 3), proponents of intervention argued that sickness damaged the economy, calculating precise examples of productive days lost. The year was 1917 and America was at war, so the importance of health to the country's military strength was also stressed.

2 In the context of the campaign the assumption of the reformers was that social insurance would lead to a reduction in productivity loss. It is implicit that state benefits will reduce sickness by speeding recovery. The emphasis on the risks of occupational diseases may have been directed particularly to employers, whose financial contribution would be crucial. The central assumption throughout is that it was the health of able, adult men that mattered.

Productivism therefore illuminates the policy context in which decisions were taken. It is also useful in explaining why America was different, because for various reasons the state may not have perceived it to be essential to intervene to make the economy more efficient. Industrial wages were higher than in Europe and workers were better able to purchase health care directly, especially if they were members of a workplace assurance fund. There was a buoyant labour market, fuelled by mass migration from Europe and elsewhere, and American productivity was surging ahead as entrepreneurs developed the continent's rich natural resources. Arguably, then, states had less impetus to propose welfare.

However, as with all explanations that tie health politics to the general development of the economy, the productivist case is somewhat unsatisfactory. While these arguments loomed large in the policy debates about the start of NHI, they featured less as the twentieth century progressed and welfare states expanded. The explanation also attributes agency to a 'ruling class' that is unproblematically assumed to be at the behest of big industrialists. Was this really a fair description of policy-making in the pluralist democracies of the West?

Politics: Democratic rights bring social rights?

In the 1950s, the sociologist T.H. Marshall argued that it was the advance of democracy itself that had opened the way for the welfare state. The key was a changing conception of citizenship. The right to vote in regular elections meant that ordinary people were no longer subjects who were ruled over, but participants in the political process. With political citizenship came 'social citizenship' – in other words, new rights to social welfare. Drawing particularly on the British case, Marshall tracked the gradual extension of the vote to working-class males in the nineteenth century, and noted (as we saw in Chapter 3) how early social reforms in public health and education had followed this expansion of the franchise. The welfare state of the twentieth century was therefore the full flowering of this new social citizenship.

Exercise 9.4 Health and party politics

The British Liberal Party issued the poster below in the year of the passage of Britain's National Health Insurance legislation. The figure on the right is David Lloyd George, then Chancellor of the Exchequer. Note that a 'Bill' is a piece of proposed legislation still to be approved by Parliament. Once you have studied the poster, answer the question that follows.

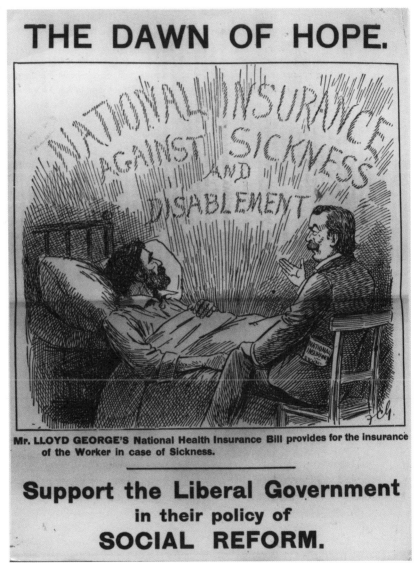

Figure 9.1 Poster, 'The Dawn of Hope', 1911
Credit: Getty Images

• Does this source provide support for Marshall's theory?

Feedback

In evaluating posters as historical sources we must be careful not to make assumptions about how viewers may have received and understood them. All they really tell us is what those who commissioned them wanted to say. Nonetheless, this early example of medical politics as party propaganda illustrates assumptions about the voter appeal of health benefits. Here is one possible interpretation:

The Liberals were urging that the intended recipients of NHI – 'the Worker' – should support their proposals, which had not yet become law. This in turn would boost their electoral chances. The image uses a religious metaphor, with the patient, like a Biblical saint, experiencing a revelatory vision. This emphasizes the symbolic potency of health in political discourse, representing a panacea for deep-seated fears about suffering and death. Meanwhile Lloyd George exudes reassurance and paternal authority, his posture at the bedside evoking that of the physician (compare this with the image of the Medical Officer of Health in Chapter 10). This was a time when public faith in the doctor was high, thanks to the aura of scientific expertise conferred by the advances in bacteriology, and the poster seeks to persuade voters that they should place the same trust in politicians.

The source therefore partly supports Marshall's theory, in that it suggests health policy was now a significant element in the relationship between politicians and people. However, the emphasis on the gains enjoyed by adult working-class males also reminds us of the productivism and legitimation arguments.

The problem with Marshall's thesis is that it relies heavily on the British case. Political rights were not very extensive in Bismarck's Germany, where the first NHI was very much a reform from above. Nor is it obvious that democratic rights inevitably led to more state welfare. The American example of the 1917 California referendum shows that genuine grassroots participation could produce the opposite result if citizens worried it would mean higher taxes.

Political culture and national character

A slightly different take on political history, advanced particularly by American commentators, is the argument that national culture shapes the health system. Here, for example, is the prominent Republican politician, Rudy Guiliani speaking in 2007:

> The American way is not single-payer, government-controlled anything. That's a European way of doing something; that's frankly a socialist way ...
>
> (Steinhauser, 2007)

Behind this lies the assumption that America's political culture sets great store on liberty and individual choice, and that this in turn arises from the historical forces that shaped its national character. A key factor often cited is the experience of settling the country, which inculcated a 'frontier spirit' of independence, self-reliance and a 'can-do' mentality.

There are two big problems with this thesis. First, Americans certainly have been ready to adopt 'government-controlled' solutions when needs arose, such as Social Security during the Depression or Medicare from the 1960s. Second, opinion poll data at various times have shown substantial proportions of the population willing to consider publicly funded social insurance. Thus the 'national character' argument should probably be understood largely as political rhetoric.

Political beliefs: Labour mobilization

Perhaps, then, we should reject vague appeals to national character or citizenship rights and look more closely at the relationship between health policy and political beliefs. One powerful version of this argument is that it was organized labour, acting either through the trade union movement or through social democratic political parties, which championed the expansion of health systems. They did this because the redistributive elements of NHI or NHS systems favoured those on lower incomes. This 'labour mobilization' thesis applies not to the beginnings of NHI, but to the subsequent reforms of the mid twentieth century that brought universal coverage and more public provision.

There were various countries where social democratic parties were in power when major health reforms took place. Sweden was one, and Britain another. Indeed, the coming of the NHS was presented at the time as a socialist measure, whose creator, Aneurin Bevan, was thoroughly working class, coming from a coal-mining family in industrial Wales and building his career through the trade union movement.

In America, we can point to the early *lack* of enthusiasm from trade unions as a possible explanation for the absence of NHI. In the 1910s, labour feared that social insurance might draw support away from the unions, which also offered health benefits, and would detract from their own campaign, the priority of which was higher wages. By the 1940s, unions concentrated on getting companies to provide health cover as part of employment benefit packages, perhaps because the chances of national political success now seemed so slim.

However, labour mobilization only offers a partial explanation. The experience in Germany under the Fascist dictatorship (1933–1945) provides a strong counter-example. Here the Bismarck system thrived as the basis for health coverage, at the same time as trade unionism was suppressed and socialists outlawed. Closer inspection of the British case also paints a more complex picture, because the White Paper that presented early proposals for the NHS was the work of a coalition government led by Conservatives. Even without Labour's victory in 1945, a comprehensive NHS with massively expanded coverage would almost certainly have come into being.

Political alliances: Solidarism

Perhaps, then, a more satisfactory explanation is that health service reform happened when the parties representing the interests of the middle classes aligned with those representing labour, to back health reform. These were moments in which, in Peter Baldwin's (1990) words, the necessary 'social solidarity' to carry forward the welfare state was forged. However, Baldwin also stresses that middle-class solidarity did not arise from humanitarianism but from self-interest. Even for those on good incomes, the costs of modern medicine are such that NHI or NHS systems can represent a better deal than commercial payment or profit-driven private insurance. Not only do state systems drive insurance prices down by expanding the risk pool, they also give governments leverage to hold down costs of drugs and services.

So, in the austerity years following the Second World War, the British NHS looked like an attractive option not just for poorer people, but for other income groups as well. And when in the 1950s and 1960s West Germany gradually expanded NHI coverage almost to universalism, this was not driven by social democratic politicians, but by conservatives representing groups like farmers and small business-people, who wanted to enjoy the same health privileges as the working class. The USA was slightly different, because there had never been a clear class divide between the political parties. However, when the Democratic Party carried through the Medicare and Medicaid reforms in the 1960s, these too arose from a broad social consensus that a limited form of NHI was desirable. The benefits of Medicare in particular, which also went to older people on middle incomes, were sufficiently attractive to defeat those familiar American arguments about liberty and individual choice.

Political structures: Institutionalism

There is one final argument advanced by political scientists that helps us to understand why major health reforms became possible at certain points, and also why their timing and nature varied from place to place. The starting point is that health system reforms are always difficult, because there are powerful vested interests that oppose them. These include employers, who resent the additional costs that fall on them, drug companies, who fear that governments will reduce their profits, and private insurers, who worry they will lose business. Above all, though, it has been doctors who have resented the incursion of the state into their territory. As Chapter 4 showed, the nineteenth century witnessed the consolidation of the profession, which rose in wealth and status, with organizations to further its interests (e.g. the American Medical Association (AMA) (1847), the British Medical Association (BMA) (1832)). The question then arises of whether a country's political institutions offer such interest groups the opportunity to block legislation, even when elected leaders are in favour.

The contrasting institutions and health politics of Britain and the United states provide an illustration. In the British system, elections have almost always delivered a straight majority of votes in Parliament to one of two main parties. The Prime Minister is also the party leader, and is therefore responsible for initiating legislation. There is a strong 'party whip', meaning that parliamentarians in the governing party are expected to vote with the government, rather than exercise independence. And although there are two 'Houses' in Parliament, the elected Commons and the unelected Lords, the 'Upper House' can only delay and amend legislation, not veto a Bill passed by the Commons. So, in Britain, if a government has a strong majority and is determined on action, as was Labour in 1945–48, it can get its way. In practice, the BMA raised strong objections to the NHS, and was granted some concessions by Bevan, like good rates of remuneration and the continuation of private medicine, but it could not stop major reform.

Now consider the political institutions of the United States. Here, there is a separation of powers and both the Congress and the Executive (the President) can initiate legislation, which may in itself be a recipe for disagreement. There is also a weak party whip, and Presidents cannot rely on the loyal support of party members in Congress. This was a key factor for mid twentieth century health reform, which was opposed by fiscally and socially conservative southern Democrats. America also has a complex legislative process, with Health Bills having to pass votes both in the House of Representatives, in different Committees of Congress, and then in the Senate, giving plenty of potential veto points for opponents. Finally, pressure groups exercise huge power over politicians, either through campaign donations or through their propaganda machines. For instance, in 1950 the AMA spent $2.25 million attacking NHI, compared with $36,000 spent by its supporters (Star, 1982, p. 287). All these institutional factors have made it harder for American Presidents who supported NHI, and had the backing of voters, to implement their policies.

Exercise 9.5 Pressure groups and health politics

The cartoon below appeared in a British newspaper at the time of the NHS Acts. The British Dental Association had threatened to boycott the NHS when the new service began, in a tussle with the government over salary levels. The character on the right is Minister of Health, Aneurin Bevan. Once you have looked at the cartoon, answer the questions that follow.

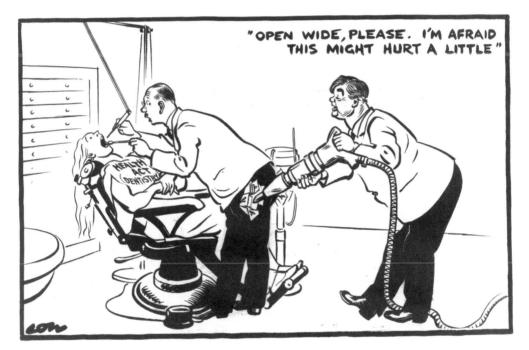

Figure 9.2 Cartoon, 'Open wide please', by David Low
Source: Evening Standard, December 1948

1 What does the image tell us about relations between government and dentists?
2 Can we draw any conclusions about public attitudes to health pressure groups?

Feedback

1 Bevan, representing the government, aims an outsize drill at the dentist's pocket, which is stuffed with money. The message is that the government is exerting its power to set the level of earnings when the NHS Act is passed, despite the dentists' objections at the 'pain' this will cause.

2 In using visual sources we must avoid drawing unfounded conclusions about what contemporary viewers might have felt. With press cartoons we must also remember that newspapers tend to have a political bias, which could influence their contents. Nonetheless, the artist presumably thought that readers would understand and respond to the joke in the cartoon because it touched popular sentiments.

The humour hinges on the apprehension we all feel about a visit to the dentist, with its promise of pain and discomfort. Here we are invited to laugh at the dentist, because now it is he who is going to 'hurt'. One reading could be that the dentist is represented unsympathetically as aloof and greedy (symbolized by the money spilling from his pocket). Bevan is drawn with a cheery smile, suggesting that he is regarded affectionately.

Although we would need to check this with other sources, a preliminary conclusion would be that public opinion sympathized with government against the medical professionals. Indeed, in the event the dentists' boycott soon fizzled out because they were not united in opposition to the NHS, which tends to support this reading.

Summary

In the course of the twentieth century, high-income countries have developed complex health systems. The state has played a dominant role, ensuring the coverage of citizens, regulating the behaviour of medical professions, and improving access and quality, either by directly providing or contracting health services. The result for most countries has been a system that combines private coverage, social insurance and state provision, with past political choices determining the nature of the mix. We must be wary of simplistic characterizations of differences between nations. For example, although it was not until 2010 that America under Barack Obama took its bitterly contested steps towards universalism, it would not be true to say its public sector was small. In fact, in 1997 public spending on health per capita in the United States (US$1643) was higher than in Britain (US$1156) (WHO, 2000, p. 195).

In this chapter, we have presented leading theories of health system development, and suggested that none alone is sufficient to explain the empirical differences (although, of course, you may disagree!). In the pluralist Western democracies, with their steadily expanding electorates, a multiplicity of motives inspired policy-makers. Sometimes bosses and governments were concerned about legitimation and economic efficiency, sometimes not, while labour movements varied in their support for health service reform, and the middle classes of Western Europe and the United States grew progressively more interested in sharing in the benefits of publicly funded provision. National political institutions were also influential, over both the shape and timing of legislation. Perhaps the only thing we can say with certainty is that social justice and an unalloyed humanitarian concern for the health of the people was rarely the dominant factor in the development of health care systems. In the following chapter we will explore other forces of change which shaped public health in the West during the first half of the twentieth century, both as discipline and practice.

References and further reading

Baldwin P (1990) *The Politics of Social Solidarity: Class Bases of the European Welfare States, 1875–1975.* Cambridge: Cambridge University Press.

Bauriedl U (1981) 100 years of German social insurance: Looking back on a century of self-managed social security, *International Social Security Review*, 34(4): 403–9.

Briggs A (1961) The welfare state in historical perspective, *European Journal of Sociology*, 2: 221–58.

Harris B (2004) *The Origins of the British Welfare State: Social Welfare in England and Wales, 1800–1945*. Basingstoke: Palgrave Macmillan.

Immergut E (1992) *Health Politics: Interests and Institutions in Western Europe*. Cambridge: Cambridge University Press.

Liberal Federation (1885) *The Radical Programme*. London: Chapman & Hall.

Light D and Schuller A (eds) (1986) *Political Values and Health Care: The German Experience*. London: MIT Press.

Marshall TH (1950) *Citizenship and Social Class, and Other Essays*. Cambridge: Cambridge University Press.

New Jersey Commission (1917) *Report on Health Insurance by the New Jersey Commission on Old Age, Insurance and Pensions*. Rahway, NJ: New Jersey Reformatory Print.

Polanyi K (2001) *The Great Transformation: The Political and Economic Origins of our Time* (2nd edn). Boston, MA: Beacon Press.

Starr P (1982) *The Social Transformation of American Medicine*. New York: Basic Books.

Steinhauser P (2007) Giuliani attacks Democratic health plans as 'socialist', *CNN.com politics*, 31 July.

World Health Organization (2000) *World Health Report 2000*. Geneva: WHO.

Public health in the twentieth century I: 1900–1945

Virginia Berridge

Overview

Public health has undergone significant changes in definition and scope over time. As we saw in Chapters 2 and 3, in the nineteenth century it initially had a strong environmental dimension and concentrated on sanitary solutions and interventions. The coming of the bacteriological 'revolution' in the late nineteenth century instigated a change within public health away from the environment and towards the role of laboratory science. In the early years of the twentieth century, a fresh reformulation took place. This laid stress on personal responsibility and on education but was also accompanied by welfare initiatives. In the inter-war years, public health practitioners redefined their role again to include the running of services. Fresh ideas came on the agenda through the new doctrine of 'social medicine'. Public health also became important globally through new international organizations.

Learning objectives

After working through this chapter, you will be able to:

- describe how the definition of public health changed between 1900 and 1945
- use primary sources to identify and explain some of the issues involved in changing definitions of public health
- assess the implications and factors involved in reformulations of public health both nationally and internationally

Key term

Disease eradication The conclusive destruction of infective reservoirs and cessation of transmission of a given disease in a population or area.

Introduction

In Chapter 2, we outlined the stages of change within public health since the eighteenth century and left the story in the later years of the nineteenth century. We now move to the first half of the twentieth century when public health began to focus on education and personal hygiene, sometimes called 'personal prevention'. New theories about the health of the population were accompanied by fears of a decline in the overall quality of the population, which affected many European and North American countries at this time. Public health changed its role again in the period between the two World Wars. There were debates about how effective its role really was and whether crucial issues of population health and nutrition were being neglected.

Exercise 10.1

'Public health' tends to be a catch-all term that means different things to different people. Moreover, public health is not unchanging: as state intervention in health issues expanded from the mid nineteenth century, public health initiatives began to operate in different ways and different public health arenas came into being.

We outline below some of the different ways in which public health operated by the beginning of the twentieth century. Using examples from your own country, write down the forms of public health that you think might fall under each heading.

1 Public health institutions
2 Public health as a profession
3 Public health as a way of thinking about health, as a form of knowledge or ideology

Feedback

1 A public health institution might be a health department either locally or nationally. It could be an agency disseminating health education, again either locally or nationally. It could be a voluntary organization promoting a health message about an issue. In Britain, for example, the central Ministry of Health was established just after the First World War in 1919.
2 A public health professional is often a medical person with a public health role. A major example is the Medical Officer of Health in the UK, or the Chief Medical Officer at the national level. Such public health professions vary over time and also in different countries. For example in the United States, public health officials did not have to be medically qualified, although this is now the case there and in the UK also.
3 Public health as a way of thinking about health incorporates some of the changes we are discussing, for example whether it focuses on the environment or the individual. The role of science, whether it was epidemiology or laboratory science, in that way of thinking has also become more important. Increasingly, too, public health has become seen as a multidisciplinary enterprise drawing on a variety of different occupations and disciplines.

Public health in the early twentieth century

Sanitary reform had delivered considerable benefits in the course of the early twentieth century with respect to water supply, sewage removal and food production.

But implementation was slow and the problem of inadequate housing remained. Some mortality rates remained high: this was particularly the case for infant mortality. As one can see from Figure 10.1, in Britain, just before 1900, infant mortality rates began to increase.

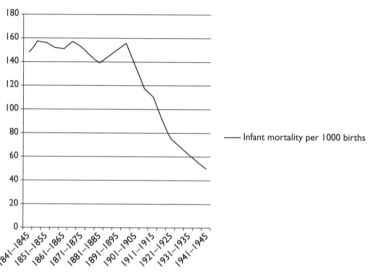

Figure 10.1 Infant mortality per 1000 births, 1841–1945

Source: Office for National Statistics (2007)

Knowledge of these statistics fuelled other concerns. Towards the end of the nineteenth century, the balance of economic power was shifting away from Britain and towards Germany and the United States. During the Boer War (1899–1902), Britain struggled to defeat the Boer farmers and this led to a period of debate and investigation of the causes of imperial decline. The examination of recruits for the army produced a devastating picture of physical inadequacy. An inter-departmental committee report on physical deterioration published in 1904 helped increase the anxieties about the quality and quantity of the population (Inter-Departmental Committee, 1904). Fears of racial decline stimulated eugenic views that advocated measures of race hygiene such as the physical segregation or even sterilization of those deemed mentally and physically unfit.

Contemporaries identified 'scourges' that could potentially decimate the race: these were tuberculosis, venereal disease and alcoholism (discussed in Chapters 6 and 7). But increasingly the debate concentrated, in Britain and elsewhere, on the health of mothers, infants and children; common objects of concern in public health. In countries such as Canada, Australia, New Zealand and Sweden, there was also growing anxiety about the health of this section of the population after 1900 (Porter, 1994). There was a debate about what was called 'national efficiency', inspired by eugenic theories that were concerned with the quality of the population. So-called 'maternal inefficiency', which stressed the role of inadequate and ignorant mothering, the role of working mothers and lack of breast-feeding or proper care, came to the fore rather than wider environmental factors. There were differing emphases among public health professionals working in government. Sir Arthur Newsholme, Medical Officer to the Local Government Board, placed most blame on women's work and also stressed poverty and environmental disadvantage. George Newman, however, a medical professional who was Medical Officer to the Board of Education, emphasized inadequate and feckless mothering (Lewis, 1980; Eyler, 1997).

Exercise 10.2

Much emphasis was thus placed on instruction for motherhood, on the provision of clinics and health visitors (discussed in Chapter 4) rather than the provision of material aid. Their role was expanded and reliance placed on their intervention in working-class homes. The extract below is from rules for health visitors in the early years of the twentieth century. Read through it and then answer the questions that follow.

> 'They must carry with them carbolic powder, explain its use, and leave it where it is accepted; direct the attention of those they visit to the evils of bad smells, want of fresh air, impurities of all kinds; give hints to mothers on feeding and clothing their children-where they find sickness assist in promoting the comfort of the⁻invalid by personal help, and report such cases to their superintendent. They must urge the importance of cleanliness, thrift and temperance on all possible occasions. They are desired to get as many as possible to join the mothers' meetings of their districts, to use all their influence to induce those they visit to attend regularly at their respective places of worship, and to send their children to school.'
>
> From 'A model Ladies Health Society' (1906), *British Medical Journal*, i: 152
> (quoted in Davies, 1988)

1 What type of advice is the health visitor offering?
2 What is the role of the health visitor in relation to sickness?
3 What sort of wider activities does the health visitor promote and what implications do you think these may have?
4 Can you think of advantages and disadvantages of the approaches outlined here?

Feedback

1 The health visitor's advice is focused on the modification of personal habits such as cleanliness, and the ways in which mothers are feeding their children.
2 The health visitor does not deal with sickness and does not offer any access to health services.
3 The health visitor is also promoting activities such as religious involvement that have a strong moral dimension. These might be considered to be beyond the bounds of health advice. Their wider concern is with ensuring that those visited are living lives in a way that conforms with dominant social norms. The group meetings suggested for mothers would also help with this.
4 *Advantages* could be that mothers who have few domestic skills or knowledge are helped to acquire these. *Disadvantages* are that the role of the health visitor does not

encompass wider social factors that might be causing ill-health or poor family hygiene. Their role also presupposes certain standards and modes of behaviour that may not be shared by the family being visited.

It is clear that infant mortality had deeper roots than simply the failings of individual mothers. In England and Wales before the First World War, infant mortality in unskilled labouring families was double that of families belonging to the upper two social classes. It is likely that social conditions as well as individual failings played a significant role. However, once again women's behaviour was blamed for public health concerns. The role of the health visitor, originally a policing one, changed, as we saw in Chapter 4, and she became more welcome in working-class families as time passed (Marks, 1996). Ultimately though health visiting was only one of several factors which brought about the fall in infant mortality illustrated in Figure 10.1. These included not only improved welfare provision, like school medical services and antenatal clinics, but also milk pasteurization, continuing investment in sanitation, the advance of female education and the adoption of family limitation.'

Public health in the inter-war years

Between the two World Wars, there were significant developments in public health. Public health operated in different ways; it stressed, as we have seen with the focus on mothers and children, *the education of individuals*. In some countries, the UK in particular, it also took over the *running of state health services*. And it also began to develop *internationally*, providing the origins of what we would now call 'global health'. We will deal with each of these aspects in turn, as well as the controversies that they have generated. These are relevant to debates in the present about the role that public health should play.

Public health as health education

Educating the public had been a function of public health since the late nineteenth century, but this function developed markedly in the inter-war years. In Britain, an avalanche of publicity about health emanated from government health departments and voluntary organizations in the 1920s and 1930s. One significant development was the new role of national organizations in this field. In Britain the Central Council for Health Education was established in 1927, based on what had been called the British Social Hygiene Council, which had originally had responsibility for education about venereal diseases. The turn of the century focus on venereal disease was broadening to encompass education of the population on other health matters.

Let us look at one example of how this operated at the local level, in Leicester in the English Midlands. The local government health committee there began to hold annual health weeks in the 1920s. It distributed handbooks and put up posters. It also screened films, had doctors and nurses giving health talks, and arranged exhibitions and tea parties for mothers and children. The local organization took part in a national health campaign in 1937 that included talks, newspaper articles and a public meeting where people listened to a radio broadcast by the Prime Minister, Neville Chamberlain (Welshman, 2000).

Exercise 10.3

Read through the leaflet below, which was issued by a local infant welfare centre in the UK during the inter-war years, and then answer the questions that follow.

HEALTHABET

A for Ambition to thrive and be wealthy.
B for the Baby that's happy if healthy.
C for the Children taught to be clean.
D for the Dirt that brings illness unseen.
E for Enjoyment that cleanliness brings.
F for the Fight against all filthy things.
G for the Germs you should wash right away.
H for the Health you improve every day.
I for Infection wherever you go.
J for the Jollity healthy folk know.
K for the Knowledge that dirt is wrong.
L for Life that is healthy and long.
M for Microbes that swarm everywhere.
N for Neglect that gives them a lair.
O for Often—to wash often is right.
P for Pride in your home clean and bright.
Q for the Quick way to banish all ill.
R for the Right way—clean with a will.
S for Sickness, in dirty homes rife.
T for Teaching a healthier life.
U for Ugliness dirt spreads about.
V for the Vigour that cleans it all out.
W for Washing—that watchword of purity.
X for eXcellent health and security.
Y for Youth—they're the Nation to-morrow.
Z for the Zeal that makes health banish sorrow.

Published by HEALTH & CLEANLINESS COUNCIL, 5, Tavistock Sq., London, W.C.1.

Figure 10.2 Healthabet
Source: Webster (1993)

1 Itemize the different ways in which the leaflet claims that health can be maintained.
2 What type of actions and activities are these? Are they comprehensive or do they leave things out?

Feedback

1 The leaflet itemizes: good personal habits, including cleanliness; a desire for self-improvement; vigorous activity; working hard; being young; information and instruction; and avoidance of dirt and infection.
2 The actions and activities itemized by the leaflet focus on self-improvement and the development of good habits. Sickness is connected with dirt and so the card focuses on what individuals can do to help themselves, rather than on the broader structural influences on health such as poor housing, poverty or unemployment.

Public health running state health services

In the inter-war years in Britain, public health doctors substantially increased their powers because they ran a widening range of services provided by local authorities. We use the case study of inter-war Britain to look at the issues that surround this type of formal public health activity. Practitioners in public health have often discussed whether it is better located within health services or in the community. Was the strategy for public health in the inter-war years of being focused on health services a good one?

By 1939, local authorities were allowed to provide: maternal and child welfare services; a school medical service; dentistry; school meals and milk; tuberculosis schemes including sanatorium treatment, clinics and aftercare; health centres; and they also had responsibility for developing local regional cancer schemes. The most important change came in 1929 when local authorities were allowed to take over the administration of the Poor Law hospitals and so many Medical Officers of Health found themselves acting in the role of medical superintendent of the local hospital. Public health doctors confidently expected that their 'empire' of services would form the basis of a national health service. However, under the NHS this did not happen.

There are two views on this period of public health activity. Some, in particular public health doctors after the Second World War, saw it as a *golden age* when the profession had great power and influence. However other historians have taken a different view and see it as a *wrong turning*. Below we look at the arguments on both sides and their implications for current public health practice. In recent times, historians have begun to take a more nuanced view, and we will look at this newer interpretation as well.

Was this a golden age?

There were many positive aspects to this era for public health. It saw a three-fold decrease in infectious disease mortality rates (from around 350 per 100,000 population in 1917, to about 150 per 100,000 in 1937, before reaching just 10–20 per 100,000 in 1957) (Office for National Statistics, 2008). Preventive and curative services, so often fragmented, were well integrated, for example in the school health service and in infant and maternal welfare. Public health was clearly identifiable as an activity at the local level. The Medical Officer of Health was a well-known local figure who worked with local politicians, and was known to the general public. The annual public health report brought together health statistics on the local area. The Medical Officer of Health headed a well-staffed department with workers ranging from health visitors to sanitary inspectors. It was easy to be responsive to the locality and to local wishes since the public health area coincided with that of local government. This was a period of expanding public provision, with greater equity and health being seen as a right of citizenship. These ideas underwent further development during the Second World War.

Was this a wrong turning?

Some historians, in particular Charles Webster and Jane Lewis, have argued that this range of activity was a wrong turning for public health. Their view is that by taking on a vast range of services without a clear view of what public health was all about, the occupation made itself vulnerable in the post-war reorganization of health services and it did not act to improve the health of the poorer sections of the population (Webster, 1982; Lewis, 1991). They point out that public health doctors were over-stretched because of their role within curative health services. There was less distinction between what they did and that of other health practitioners. In particular, the respective activities of the general practitioner and the Medical Officer of Health seemed to overlap.

Sir William Savage, Medical Officer of Health for Somerset, speaking in 1935, deplored the impact of the expansion of services on public health. Savage was near retirement and wanted to focus on the traditional sanitary aspects of public health activity.

> We have become administrators of beds largely occupied by the end product of disease and supervisors of defectives [under mental health illness legislation]; in a word, largely enmeshed in functions which are not our proper business.
>
> (quoted in Lewis, 1991, p. 209)

Jane Lewis has highlighted the example of diphtheria immunization to support the 'wrong turning' argument. Effective immunization agents were available by the early 1920s and there were reports of successful trials in Canada and the United States. The British public health profession were responsible for immunization campaigns at the local level, but remained distrustful of this approach. Many concentrated their efforts on swabbing throats and noses to identify carriers and on confining victims in hospital. This meant that the death rate in Canada fell in the 1920s and 1930s whereas in Britain there was no decline until 1941, when a national immunization scheme was implemented (Lewis, 1986).

In general, public health doctors favoured the continuance of expensive institutional solutions in these years, including for tuberculosis, and they paid much less attention to their preventive role or that of 'community watchdog'. The case of diphtheria reflects this problem, as did the concern about the effect of long-term unemployment on nutritional standards and mortality and morbidity rates. The historian Charles Webster argued that most Medical Officers of Health filed optimistic annual reports about the health of their communities. They told the Ministry of Health at the centre what it wanted to hear.

Nutrition and malnutrition

During the 1930s, the lead in raising questions about the health status of the population was thus taken not by public health professionals, but by political lobbying groups, such as the Children's Minimum Council, the Committee against Malnutrition and the National Unemployed Workers' Movement, all of which called for a higher level of unemployment benefit to enable families to secure minimal nutritional requirements. A social scientist, Richard Titmuss, undertook a survey of infant mortality and concluded that a decline in the infant mortality rate was not accompanied by a narrowing of the gap between the social classes. A small number of consultants, in particular obstetricians and gynaecologists, also drew attention to high maternal mortality and morbidity rates. A new scientific discipline, nutrition, appeared on the scene. In *Food Health and Income* (1936), John Boyd Orr showed that one-tenth of the population and one-fifth of children were ill nourished.

One of the few public health doctors to draw attention to the interconnection between unemployment and health was G.C.M. McGonigle, the Medical Officer of Health for Stockton on Tees. In *Poverty and Public Health*, McGonigle and Kirby (1936) reported that the death rate among the poorer sections of the local population was twice that of more affluent families.

This pessimistic historical interpretation of inter-war public health implies that public health could have played a greater role in advancing social justice in this time of high unemployment. Some historians have recently challenged this view, arguing that there was considerable local variety in the funding allocated to public health. Analysis of expenditure on public health locally shows that some areas increased their spending in the inter-war years (Levene, Powell and Stewart, 2004). There was an improvement in infant mortality even though maternal mortality remained high. This newer historical interpretation argues that running services was not a diversion for public health. Rather, it started to bring together preventive and curative services. The influence of a high-profile local official, the Medical Officer of Health, could be considerable and tells us about the role of personal leadership in public health (Gorsky, 2008).

Exercise 10.4

Figure 10.3 shows a picture of a Medical Officer of Health, illustrating the activities under his control at the local level. Look at the picture and then answer the questions that follow.

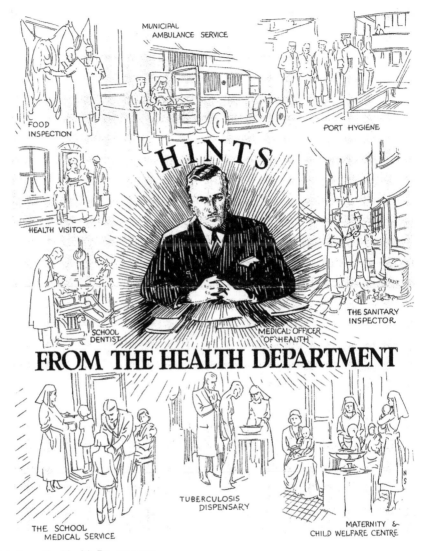

Figure 10.3 Hints from the Health Department

Source: Wellcome Library

1 What does the picture illustrate about the role of the Medical Officer of Health?
2 Itemize what you see as the advantages and disadvantages of the role of the Medical Officer of Health as portrayed in this picture.

Feedback

1 The Medical Officer of Health is in charge of a wide range of services and operates as a 'health department'. Both curative and preventive activities (for example, with infant welfare) come under his umbrella.

2 *Advantages* include: the Medical Officer of Health as a recognizable figure in the community responsible for its health; the integration of services for treatment and prevention of ill-health; the possibility of bringing together a wide range of health and other professionals; the ability to respond to local needs and circumstances. *Disadvantages* include: a focus on services rather than other interventions; an inability to examine or deal with the effects of poverty and poor diet or housing, which also have an impact on health; a local response that may not be replicated in other areas of need.

Public health at the international level

This national and local case study illustrates some of the dilemmas in the role of public health and the ways in which it defined itself. However, public health did not only operate at these levels. Increasingly, it was also an international enterprise and this aspect began to come to the fore in the 1920s and 1930s.

The international aspects of public health activity dated back to the nineteenth century. The period from the Congress of Vienna (1815) to the outbreak of war in 1914 saw the emergence of wide-ranging international cooperation in many areas: law, economics, labour, religious and intellectual movements, social and welfare organizations, and humanitarian causes. International sanitary conferences began to be held, but disputes concerning the aetiology of diseases such as cholera bedevilled many of the early meetings. Scientific developments, such as Snow's work in London and Koch's in Germany, had no impact on the conferences that followed these discoveries (1859 and 1885 respectively). However, effective cooperation in areas of science and medicine did make progress through the century, which initially took the form of international congresses on specific areas, for example the first statistical congress (1853), the first congress of ophthalmologists (1857) and the first congress of chemists (1860). Many of these went on to form international committees and associations. The statistical congress of 1853 initiated the preparation of a nomenclature of the causes of death that would be applicable to all countries. This was adopted and revised at subsequent meetings and taken forward by the International Statistical Institute formed in 1890. At the close of the century, the momentum for cooperation between non-state actors, and later between states, focused on the exchange of information, and represented the first moves towards an international vocabulary (standards, classification) in medicine and science (Berridge, Loughlin and Herring, 2009).

The social, religious and humanitarian movements that emerged in the nineteenth century were more complex and diverse in their development. Many were characterized by popular support, but there was also a pattern of conferences leading to more permanent committees or organizations. A burgeoning middle class and the spread of evangelical religion supported many of the activities, whereas the shared experience of industrialization and urbanization spawned common social problems across a number of states. The first of four International Congresses of Charities, Correction and Philanthropy met in Brussels in 1865. These were followed in 1869 by a new series of international congresses on public and private charity that met at irregular intervals up to 1914. These meetings were attended by representatives of a wide range of philanthropic organizations and the discussions covered a broad spectrum of issues: food production, alcoholism, prison conditions, medical assistance to the poor, rehabilitation, infant mortality and the protection of women and girls (Lyons, 1963). In 1900, an international committee was formed and a bureau of information and studies followed in

1907. This 'umbrella' association emphasized the need for information exchange and an increasing number of governments sent representatives to its conferences.

A number of international 'single-issue' reform movements also came to the fore, a development seen as early as 1840 with the International Anti-Slavery Conference and later the International Committee of the Red Cross (1864). In the health and welfare field these associations could be popular in orientation or focused on specialist expertise. Some, such as the congresses on alcohol, and the resultant International Temperance Bureau (1906), mingled both activism and science (Bruun, Pan and Rexed, 1975), as did the international Central Bureau for the Campaign against Tuberculosis (1902), which emerged from a series of international conferences dating back to the 1860s. Initial activity by non-state actors in the international arena led to greater inter-governmental involvement. Many of these movements were characterized by a mix of governmental, voluntary and local activity, such as the policing on conventions around the 'white slave trade', which stemmed from the 1899 International Bureau for the Suppression of Traffic in Women and Children.

The inter-war period

In the inter-war years, matters moved further on the international scene. These decades were characterized by two interrelated developments:

1 The rise of a new style of international corporate philanthropy, in particular that developed by the Rockefeller Foundation.
2 The establishment of permanent international organizations, characterized by the League of Nations and its health organization.

The role of American foundations

The years between 1901 and 1913 witnessed the coming into being of a new form of philanthropy, characterized by the Rockefeller Foundation and other largely American institutions – the Milbank Memorial Fund, Commonwealth Fund and Sage Foundation. This new form of philanthropy developed a research-oriented view of social improvement and introduced a wider, international dimension to research and sponsorship activities, especially in the area of science and medicine. As discussed in Chapter 5, the Rockefeller Foundation had begun its health work in the eradication of hookworm in the southern United States in the early years of the twentieth century. It then developed this interest on the international stage, establishing its own initiatives through its International Health Commission (1913) and through support for clinics, training schemes, schools of public health and laboratory services throughout the world. Importantly, the Rockefeller Foundation pursued a much more interventionist programme than the US government was willing to contemplate at the time. For example, the Foundation backed the League of Nations Health Organization, even though the United States was not a member of the League. For some historians, however, the Rockefeller Foundation was a stalking horse for wider American political interests, and a central agent of biomedical imperialism, exporting a US model of public health across the world. Undoubtedly, US political interests were furthered by Rockefeller Foundation involvement in the League of Nations and through its programmes, for example, in the Far East and in Latin America. According to the historian James Gillespie, 'There was no simple imposition of an American model on compliant local populations' but 'a complicated process of bargaining and compromise [that] led to local interests dominating the

LIVERPOOL JOHN MOORES UNIVERSITY
LEARNING SERVICES

implementation of the Rockefeller programme' (Gillespie, 1995). Moreover, Paul Weindling (1995) emphasizes the relative freedom of the American foundations, as they were without public or political constraints and had no need to placate the interests of the medical profession. For example, in the aftermath of the First World War, Rockefeller Foundation support helped develop a system of socialized primary health care in Serbia, and contributed to primary health care initiatives in the United States and abroad. This relative freedom also enabled the foundations to support 'unpopular' health issues: the Rockefeller Foundation provided backing for child guidance and mental hygiene, and the Commonwealth Fund targeted mental health during the inter-war period.

Exercise 10.5

The picture below shows the operations of the International Health Commission of the Rockefeller Foundation in 1916. Look at the map and then answer the questions that follow.

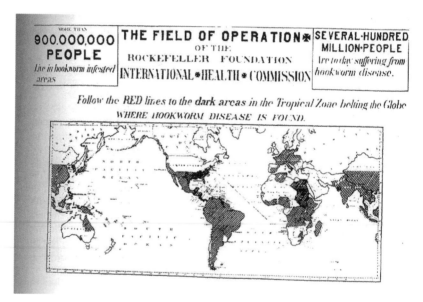

Figure 10.4 Field of operations of the International Health Commission, 1916
© Rockefeller Archive Centre
Scanned from Webster (1993, p. 114)

1 What strikes you about the geographical range of activities of the Commission?
2 What is the disease that most concerns the work of the Commission?

Feedback

1 The Commission's work is worldwide: North America, Europe, Africa and Europe.
2 There is a particular focus on hookworm based on the initial campaigns in Mexico and the southern states of America.

Through its focus on training and institution building, the Rockefeller Foundation was fundamental in creating an international network of public health experts. Drawing on the universalism of science, the Foundation emphasized technology transfer and the exchange of trained personnel. During the inter-war period, instruments developed in America to measure community health performance were transferred to Europe via the Rockefeller Foundation (Murard, 2005). Some historians have criticized this approach because it gave primacy to professionalized, increasingly technocratic solutions to public health. For example, the Rockefeller Foundation's disease eradication campaigns in Latin America became increasingly laboratory based, and there was a similar trajectory in Australia and the Pacific Islands. Historians have discussed the interpretation of the role of American foundations in international health during a period of US political isolationism – was it benign philanthropy or American imperialism by private means?

International health and the League of Nations

The Treaty of Versailles, which sealed the end of the First World War, brought into being a new organization at an international level, the League of Nations. The League had technical agencies with responsibility for health. The technical agencies of the League of Nations were its Health Organization and the International Labour Office (ILO). Initially, the ILO had an expansive vision of its role in health and welfare, legitimized by the Treaty of Versailles, which assigned it the role of protecting 'the worker against sickness, disease and injury arising out of his [sic] employment'. But the broad vision was restricted early on. Weindling comments, 'in seeking to justify its reformist demands in the universalist terms of science, it had to devolve initiatives to scientific experts whose empirically based approaches were necessarily limited to what could be proven in the laboratory' (Weindling, 1995, p. 139). Consequently, the focus of the ILO became overly technical, anchored around the production of scientific evidence of the health effects of particular hazards. Moreover, despite its overall premise that welfare was determined by socio-economic conditions, no attempt was made to correlate economic trends with the mortality and morbidity data in its labour statistics.

The League of Nations Health Organization (LNHO), the agency with responsibility for public health and social medicine, showed a similar narrowing of focus, signalled by its separation from the Social Section in 1920. The primary concern of the LNHO in the 1920s was the scientific universalism of standard setting, in terms of biological and morbidity/mortality statistics. Indeed, by 1937 approximately 72 per cent of the world's population was covered by LNHO statistics. This emphasis on international standards did, however, provide leverage for broader health debates during the economic depression of the 1930s. The LNHO developed cooperative programmes with the ILO that focused on developing social medicine on economic bases – how diet, housing and economic conditions shaped health was a key area of research. Scientific expertise served radical reform in areas like nutrition, as British scientists criticized their government by invoking nutrition standards endorsed by the LNHO/ILO – forcing them to raise the minimum standards used in calculating unemployment and maternity benefits. The existence of the organization and its work helped in transferring ideas about health and social welfare from the United States to European countries in these years.

'Unpopular issues' such as sexually transmitted infections were championed by voluntary initiatives and kept at a distance from arenas dominated by state actors. It has already been noted that the Rockefeller Foundation did provide support for mental health initiatives, whereas the ILO focused primarily on economically productive sectors of the population (not older people, the disabled or mentally ill), and the LNHO avoided the politically controversial issue of birth control. As we saw in Chapter 7, in one case, that of illicit drugs, a separate system emphasizing control of trade (although in the interests of health) was set up in the inter-war period. A series of international conventions following the Geneva Convention (1925) established and extended an import certificate system together with limitation of manufacture (Berridge, 2001).

Exercise 10.6

The relationship between corporate philanthropy and the League of Nations is under-lined by the quotation below from an historian of the League. Read the quotation and then answer the questions that follow.

'The RF [Rockefeller Foundation] helped Rajchman [the League's medical director] recruit staff; awarded travel grants to individuals visiting Geneva; recommended per-sons for expert bodies; made its own staff available for special purposes; helped assess requests for technical assistance; provided additional help to governments receiving LN [League of Nations] assistance; and funded its own schools, laboratories and insti-tutes of persons engaged in the LNHO.'

(Dubin, 1995, p. 72)

1 What do you see as the likely implications of this type of relationship?
2 Can you think of any similar relationships at the international level in the present day?

Feedback

1 The advantages of such a relationship could include a regular source of funding. However, reliance on funding could also lead to a distortion of strategy and priorities that might be made to fit those of the corporate sponsor. In this case, it has been argued that the close relationship between the Rockefeller Foundation and the League of Nations led to an emphasis on biomedical rather than social solutions to health problems.
2 There are parallels in this historic relationship with current discussions about the role of corporate philanthropy and the international organizations such as the World Health Organization and the World Bank. The historical relationships are similar to what are now called public–private partnerships in health. The dominance of the biomedical paradigm then internationally is mirrored in today's criticisms of reliance on technical solutions such as vaccination.

Social medicine

A new way of thinking about public health also came onto the agenda of some coun-tries and on the international scene in the inter-war years. Out of social hygiene ideas came novel ways of thinking about the relationships between medical and social factors and attempts to integrate ideas about prevention and cure. These became known as 'social medicine', a term still used within contemporary public health circles.

A key influence was the way in which health and medicine developed in the Soviet Union after the 1917 revolution. Social hygiene departments were set up in Russian universities and the training of doctors was based on those principles. Different trends in Russian history fed into the new understanding of health. For the Marxists, ill-health and disease were expressions of socio-economic inequality. But there was also a tradition from the time of the Tsars of understanding the social influences on disease. Both groups believed that the improvement of material conditions would result in lower disease and death rates (Solomon, 1994; Porter, 1999). In both Europe and the United States, there were attempts to create a new academic discipline of social medicine. The movement was strong in France and in Belgium. In the latter, the Rockefeller Foundation funded a chair of social medicine taken up by the social medicine pioneer René Sand in 1945. He had been developing new ideas about prevention since the 1930s, trying to integrate the principles of social medicine into what he called 'the human economy'.

There were also earlier attempts to establish social medicine in the United States and in Britain. At Yale University in the 1930s, an Institute of Human Relations was founded that tried to bring medicine and social issues together. Its leaders believed that medicine had lost sight of the fact that individuals were biological and social beings. In Britain, an Institute of Social Medicine was established at Oxford University in 1942, and moves were made to make this the dominant approach in medical training after the war. John Ryle, the first professor of social medicine at Oxford, wrote that health was the 'whole economic, nutritional, occupational, educational and psychological opportunity or experience of the individual or community'. It was confidently expected that such ideas might form the basis of public health in the post-war world.

Summary

In the first half of the twentieth century, public health changed significantly from the nineteenth-century emphasis on sanitation and the environment. It emphasized the role of personal responsibility, in particular that of mothers for the future quality of the population. In the inter-war years, the example of Britain shows some of the tensions within public health. Public health professionals were running services and distributing health education. They have been criticized by historians for paying less attention to the wider social determinants of health. But, the emergence of the new doctrine of 'social medicine' implied a further reorientation of the role of public health to encompass both medical and social dimensions. Public health also developed an important role internationally through the activities of the League of Nations and corporate philanthropy, something we investigate in more detail in the next chapter.

References and further reading

Berridge V (2001) Illicit drugs and internationalism; the forgotten dimension, *Medical History*, 45: 282–8.

Berridge V, Loughlin K and Herring R (2009) Historical dimensions of global health governance, in Buse K, Hein W and Drager N (eds) *Making Sense of Global Health Governance: A Policy Perspective* (pp. 28–46). Basingstoke: Palgrave Macmillan.

Boyd Orr J (1936) *Food, Health and Income*. London: Macmillan.

Bruun K, Pan L and Rexed I (1975) *The Gentleman's Club: International Control of Drugs and Alcohol*. Chicago, IL: University of Chicago Press.

Davies C (1988) The health visitor as mother's friend, *Social History of Medicine*, 1(1): 39–59.

Dubin M (1995) The League of Nations Health Organisation, in Weindling P (ed) *International Health Organisations and Movements, 1918–1939* (pp. 56–80). Cambridge: Cambridge University Press.

Eyler J (1997) *Sir Arthur Newsholme and State Medicine, 1885–1935*. Cambridge: Cambridge University Press.

Gillespie J (1995) The Rockefeller Foundation and colonial medicine in the Pacific, 1911–1929, in Bryder L and Dow D (eds) *New Countries and Old Medicine* (pp. 380–6). Auckland, NZ: Pyramid Press.

Gorsky M (2008) Public health in interwar England and Wales: did it fail?, *Dynamis*, 28: 175–98.

Inter-Departmental Committee on Human Deterioration (1904) *Report on the Inter-Departmental Committee on Physical Deterioration*. London: Printed for H.M. Stationery Office by Wyman & Sons.

Levene A, Powell M and Stewart J (2004) Patterns of municipal health expenditure in interwar England and Wales, *Bulletin of the History of Medicine*, 78(3): 635–69.

Lewis J (1980) *The Politics of Motherhood: Child and Maternal Welfare in England, 1900–1939*. London: Croom Helm.

Lewis J (1986) The prevention of diphtheria in Canada and Britain, 1914–1945, *Journal of Social History*, 20(1): 163–76.

Lewis J (1991) The public's health: Philosophy and practice in Britain in the twentieth century, in Fee E and Acheson RM (eds) *A History of Education in Public Health: Health that Mocks the Doctor's Rules* (pp. 194–229). Oxford: Oxford University Press.

Lyons FSL (1963) *Internationalism in Europe, 1815–1914*. Leiden: AW Sythoff.

Marks L (1996) *Metropolitan Maternity: Maternal and Infant Welfare in Early Twentieth Century London*. Amsterdam: Rodopi.

McGonigle G and Kirby J (1936) *Poverty and Public Health*. London: Victor Gollancz.

Murard L (2005) Atlantic crossings in the measurement of health: From US appraisal forms to the League of Nations health indices, in Berridge V and Loughlin K (eds) *Medicine, the Market and the Mass Media* (pp. 19–54). London: Routledge.

Office for National Statistics (2007) *Mortality Statistics: Review of the Registrar General on Deaths in England and Wales, 2005*. London: HMSO.

Office for National Statistics (2008) *Age-standardised Mortality Rates by Broad Cause and Sex, England and Wales, 1917–2007*. London: HMSO.

Porter D. (ed) (1994) *The History of Public Health and the Modern State*. Amsterdam: Rodopi.

Porter D (1999) *Health, Civilisation and the State: A History of Public Health from Ancient to Modern Times*. London: Routledge.

Reid A (2001) Health visitors and child health: Did health visitors have an impact?, *Annales de démographie historique*, 101(1): 117–37.

Solomon SG (1994) The expert and the state in Russian public health: Continuities and changes across the revolutionary divide, in Porter D (ed) *The History of Public Health and the Modern State* (pp. 183–223). Amsterdam: Rodopi.

Webster C (1982) Healthy or hungry thirties?, *History Workshop Journal*, 13(1): 110–29.

Webster C (ed) (1993) *Caring for Health: History and Diversity*. Buckingham: Open University Press.

Weindling P (ed) (1995) *International Health Organisations and Movements, 1918–1939*. Cambridge: Cambridge University Press.

Welshman J (2000) *Municipal Medicine: Public Health in Twentieth Century Britain*. Oxford: Peter Lang.

Global health

John Manton

Overview

This chapter describes the emergence of new organizational patterns in international public health since 1945, and the ways in which persistent global inequality, colonial models of disease control, and medical planning continued to shape post-colonial health care. We examine the development of primary health care as a means of managing scarce resources and poor health infrastructural coverage in the global South, as well as the changing causes and perceptions of famine. We conclude with a discussion of emerging diseases and resurgent food crises in the 1990s and 2000s.

Learning objectives

After working through this chapter, you will be able to:

- describe the impact of decolonization, conflict, access to food and economic crises on population health indicators in the global South
- use primary sources to identify and explain some of the factors shaping elements of historical continuity and change in the international organization of public health
- outline reasons for the success or failure of particular types of global health intervention over the past sixty years

Key terms

Decolonization The process of imperial withdrawal from direct rule over the former colonial territories of Africa and Asia, beginning with Indian independence in 1947, and ending with the creation of Zimbabwe in 1980. The term 'decolonization' is commonly used to designate the imperial and metropolitan processes relating to the end of direct rule, as opposed to nationalist or anti-colonial struggles for independence.

Disease elimination A reduction of the prevalence of a disease to a level at which it is no longer considered a substantive threat to public health. In the case of the Leprosy Elimination Strategy (1991–2000), this was taken to be less than one case per 10,000 per annum.

Globalization A process that gathered pace in the late twentieth century that underpinned expansion of industrial and trading interests and was also applied to the analysis of health issues. This stressed the definition of health issues at a level that transcended national boundaries and even the remit of the established international bodies such as the World Health Organization, and believed that the interconnectedness of such issues was greater than ever before.

Political economy of health A field of enquiry that seeks to understand the structural relations between global political and economic processes and regional disparities in health indicators. In doing so, it critically examines strategies for effecting and preventing solutions to structural inequalities.

Post-colonial Pertaining to the politics, society and culture of newly independent states.

Treponemal diseases A group of diseases caused by subspecies of *Treponema pallidum*. These include non-venereal endemic syphilis (bejel), pinta, childhood syphilis and yaws, as well as venereal syphilis.

Introduction

In terms of expenditure on health and sanitation, and of ideological and scientific arguments shaping the field of public health, the significance of the economically dominant European and North American national powers is clearly signalled throughout this book. The stories of tropical medicine and global health trace the relationship between the needs and priorities of the industrial nations of the global North and the health of people whose economic lives seemed marginal to the growth of global wealth. At times, as in the case of twentieth-century Brazil, economic development, large-scale poverty and a climate favourable to the spread of infectious disease existed alongside one another. Across large swathes of the globe, medical research and the coordination of public health services relied on substantial transfers of funding and expertise from industrialized nations.

Many of the hallmarks of colonial and early twentieth century public health were echoed during and beyond the era of decolonization. However, the major developments in the realm of global health in the second half of the twentieth century centred around (1) the realignment of international public health strategies under the direction of bodies such as the World Health Organization (WHO), and (2) the emergence of a new political economy of health dominated by expatriate technical advisory networks and the development of primary health care systems. This chapter describes the emergence of new international public health bodies, and notes some of the problems of poverty and health they faced. It outlines successes and difficulties in disease control and the importance of nutrition and economic development in securing better health for the world's population.

Organizational change in international public health

As we saw in the previous chapter, from the later years of the nineteenth century a range of international efforts to coordinate port sanitation and quarantine, the spread of epidemic disease and transnational public health proliferated among the major trading and industrial powers. During the early decades of the twentieth century, organizations such as the Rockefeller Foundation, the League of Nations Health Organization (LNHO) and the International Labour Organization (ILO) formed part of an emerging vision of international public health. The LNHO survived the Second World War, and maintained a presence at the first World Health Assembly held in Geneva in 1948. It subsequently merged with the United Nations Relief and Rehabilitation Administration (one of a number of UN agencies initially founded to deal with post-war relief and repatriation of refugees in Europe) and the Office Internationale d'Hygiène Publique to form the core of the inter-governmental World Health Organization (WHO), which emerged from the Assembly. Between 1949 and 1956, the Soviet Union and communist allies did not take part in the running or funding of the organization (as with other UN agencies); yet, it was the first extra-continental public health organization to secure the contribution of the United States. This was both a boost to WHO's success, and an important factor in its policy development, which focused on technical interventions aimed at improving medical capacity and health planning in member countries, but excluded direct funding of health infrastructure. The WHO greatly increased technical and planning capacity in international public health. Specifically, the technical assistance model favoured by WHO in the 1960s, evident in its narrow remit for the global eradication of malaria (see Chapter 8), marked a retreat from the roots of the organization in social medicine.

Exercise 11.1

Describe the impact on your country of the World Health Organization, or another named international or expatriate non-governmental organization concerned with health or medicine. You may consider, for example, what types of projects these organizations initiated, and what their objectives and outcomes were. You may answer with reference to personal experience in the health sector.

Feedback

Everyone's answer to this question will be different! You may have identified eradication programmes sponsored by the WHO. With the WHO unable to commit to the funding of public health infrastructure, a wide variety of non-governmental bodies responded to the training, funding and supply needs of newly independent nations in the global South. Some of these agencies were global in scope: you may have mentioned one of these in your answer. The United Nations Children's Fund (UNICEF) provided material funding for many disease control programmes, while the Food and Agriculture Organization (FAO) – especially in the guise of its Freedom from Hunger campaign in the early 1960s – promoted the assessment of nutritional needs and appropriate national agricultural policies, pursued in South and Southeast Asia as 'Green Revolution' programmes for the technical improvement of agricultural production.

There are many other examples of expatriate organizations involved in global health care. Christian churches and other religious groups ran high-profile hospital networks throughout the industrial and developing world. The Rockefeller Foundation promoted activities in child health research across Asia and Africa throughout the 1960s, while Oxfam, the International Committee of the Red Cross, and new organizations such as Médecins sans Frontières became increasingly involved with global emergency humanitarian aid.

Before we examine the international public health strategies pursued by WHO and allied bodies, let us pause to consider some of the impacts of imperialism on the life and health of colonial subjects. This discussion will initially focus on some of the most egregious features of the African colonial experience, leading on to a consideration of post-war international disease control programmes and their impact on the global burden of disease.

From imperial to global health: Inequality, race, morality and health

During the twentieth century, colonial economic life became increasingly diversified, and the health problems experienced in relation to poverty and inequality were also transformed. Cities grew and urban infrastructures came increasingly under pressure; rights to live and work in the city became ever more fiercely contested. The ambiguous and highly visible nature of certain skin conditions and sexually transmitted diseases was often racialized in the fraught politics of urban colonial public health. Specifically, the confusion of endemic syphilis, yaws and sexually transmitted syphilis, diseases identified as caused by similar treponematoses, frequently led to the application of sexual health legislation as a technique of urban disease control (Vaughan, 1992).

In Kenya and apartheid South Africa, the right of permanent urban residency for African families was greatly circumscribed. In both cases, the control of African labour was theoretically based on the separation of the male urban labourer from the rural family. This was formalized in South Africa by a series of pass laws and the creation of nominally independent African homelands. In Kenya, however, where formal measures were less strict and informal structural pressures more significant, the lack of clear urban residency rights for demobilized soldiers in post-1945 Nairobi also raised economic and generational tensions in politically significant ways. This contributed in part to the rise of anti-colonial land rights struggles, epitomised by Mau Mau in the 1950s.

The ramifications for urban health in East and Southern Africa were complex. On the one hand, entrenched conditions of poverty, resulting from wage levels set deliberately below the cost of maintaining a family, and underinvestment in occupational and public health services in African areas of cities, left workers with little scope or ability to attend to their own health needs. The growth of traditional medical practices and markets in urban Southern Africa is a testament to this process. On the other hand, the very informality of settlements, quarters and services for African urban workers gave rise to informal economies centred on brewing and prostitution, providing employment for women, but also making female presence in settlements and camps a public order and a public health problem (White, 1990).

For Africans living in rural areas across much of East, Central and Southern Africa, reliance on urban wage labour to meet the costs of taxation also caused significant disruption. Households were disrupted by the need for men to engage in long-distance seasonal migration, leaving women responsible for the entirety of the burden of subsistence farming and family care. The pattern of migration – from rural Nyasaland (Malawi), Rhodesia and South Africa to the Northern Rhodesian (Zambian) Copper Belt and the South African Rand – was widely understood to have facilitated the transmission of diseases associated with urban life (such as tuberculosis and venereal syphilis), foreshadowing later concerns with the role of mass transportation in the spread of sexually transmitted diseases such as HIV/AIDS. While the African role in the transmission of these diseases and, consequently, aspects of African behaviour and sexuality, was typically highlighted by colonial observers, the impact of racist social policy and the systemic reliance of settler colonial and apartheid states on factoring the costs of the reproduction of labour out of wage equations were far more invidious factors in the mismanagement of colonial sexual health.

New weapons and programmes in disease control

The battle against epidemic treponematoses took an overtly moral and implicitly racial tone in Southern and Eastern Africa. However, elsewhere the same diseases prompted some of the first major international collaborations between new United Nations agencies concerned with human health. An early collaboration between the WHO and UNICEF in 1948 focused on controlling endemic syphilis in the difficult economic and political circumstances of post-1945 Bosnia. The success of this technical intervention relied on a series of chemotherapeutic innovations avidly pursued by medical researchers during the Second World War. The mass production of penicillin was a crucial component of this and subsequent mass campaigns against endemic treponematoses, beginning with major programmes in Haiti and Indonesia. These programmes refined methods of record-keeping and rural outreach in public health, which were subsequently applied in the global yaws control programme of 1952–1964, which treated upwards of 50 million people with one injection of long-acting penicillin. By 1965, 300 million people had been examined in 46 countries, and global prevalence reduced by 95 per cent (WHO, 2008).

The charge of optimism experienced by collaborators on major post-war disease control and eradication programmes depended crucially on new families of antibiotics and pesticides. Alongside penicillin and related antibiotics, pesticides such as DDT, and sulphone and sulphonamide drugs were widely trialled and applied in these programmes. The most famous of the post-war and independence era programmes were undoubtedly the Global Malaria Eradication Campaign (1955–1962) (see Chapter 8) and the Smallpox Eradication Campaign (1967–1979). Other significant campaigns included: the Onchocerciasis Control Programme (1974–2002) in eleven West African countries, which achieved a large measure of success in interrupting transmission of onchocerciasis (also known as river blindness); the Leprosy Elimination Strategy (1991–2000), which sought to eliminate leprosy as a public health problem (without eliminating the disease) and, more controversially, the Schistosomiasis Control Programme in Egypt, which has been associated with a rise in the prevalence of hepatitis C in the Egyptian rural population.

Exercise 11.2

The diagram below exemplifies the mobile health teams that were a central feature of many major disease control, elimination and eradication campaigns in the global South during the 1950s and 1960s. Teams such as these were responsible for the compilation of epidemiological data and the extension of health services to areas of the developing world. Often, diseases other than those for which the teams were constituted were seen at examination by the mobile team, and treated or referred. Examine the diagram carefully and answer the questions that follow.

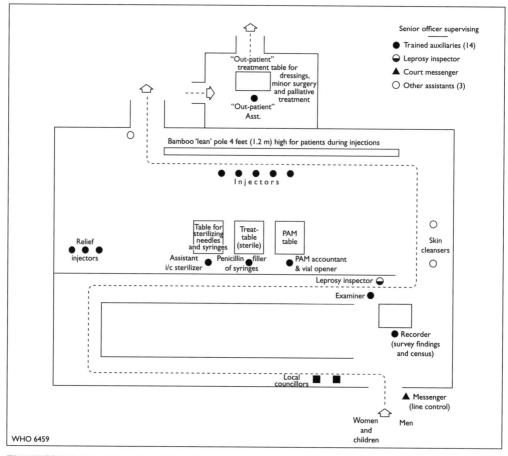

Figure 11.1 Layout of working place of yaws eradication team
Source: Zahra (1956)

1 What do you think the roles and backgrounds were of each of the different categories of workers in this diagram? What benefit might there have been to having local people in this team?
2 Where are data on the people passing through this workplace being collected and to what uses could these data be put?

Feedback

1 It would seem that the messenger, strategically placed at the point where the line enters the mobile medical complex, is understood by medical planners to be able to exert authority over those to be examined. One can assume that local councillors would be in a position to determine whether families or individuals were missing, although what their power of sanction might be we cannot be sure. It is likely that

the auxiliary assistants, perhaps the leprosy inspector, and almost certainly the skin cleansers were of local or near-local origin.

2 Data of one sort or another were assembled throughout the examination process. From local councillors to the survey recorder and leprosy inspector, through to the accountant and syringe filler and finally the outpatient assistant, information regarding the physical condition and medical needs of the processed population was gathered. Both the leprosy inspector and the outpatient assistant were concerned with issues of referral and follow-up, while the collation and tallying of population records, epidemiological data and medical ordnance requirements occupied the remainder of the staff concerned with record-keeping.

Leprosy control: From segregation to rehabilitation

Other approaches to disease control were exemplified by the attempt to deal with leprosy. While many of the impacts of colonial rule had unexpected and troubling consequences for gender relations in rural communities, not least taxation and labour recruitment, these were especially legible in the large-scale institutional apparatus arising around the project of leprosy control. The modelling and remaking of family and sexuality was not confined to the city, or to the urban–rural axis. Perhaps nowhere was this process more invasively pursued than in the mid twentieth century leprosarium.

The historian Warwick Anderson demonstrated how the island leprosarium of Culion in the US colonial Philippines gave rise to new forms of citizenship (Anderson, 2006), where the process of diagnosis, removal and incarceration generated a population that could be modelled according to visions of colonial modernity and propriety. Within leprosaria such as that at Culion, substantial clinical and research expertise in leprosy grew uncomfortably alongside confinement and segregation.

Following Filipino and Indian independence, in 1946 and 1947 respectively, significant capacity for research into the treatment and rehabilitation of leprosy patients passed out of Imperial hands. Indian leprologists, often motivated by Gandhian ideals, maintained a high profile in leprosy research after independence. These explicitly anti-colonial and self-help ideals chimed well with shifts in the treatment of leprosy that accompanied the chemotherapeutic revolution of the 1930s and 1940s. The international coordination of leprosy control substantially predated either the LNHO or the WHO. By the 1940s and 1950s, this coordination was sufficiently well advanced to be able to mandate treatment regimens, research guidelines and the dismantling of large-scale leprosaria in favour of outreach clinics and outpatient treatment.

Leprosaria did not wither away entirely, remaining as training and rehabilitation centres and as sanctuaries for the most disabled former patients. The centralization of leprosy control became less appealing during the 1960s, research capacity in leprosy diminished, and new research strategies needed to be developed to engage with more widely dispersed patient populations.

Re-emerging and new disease threats

If leprosy control offers a paradoxical vision of disease control, then the recurrence of malaria in areas where its eradication had seemed successful constitutes a tragedy of disease control. Failures of vigilance, coverage and funding, and a mixture of un-integrated spending and chronic under-investment in public health has led to the re-emergence of diseases. Alongside the resurgence of malaria in areas of successful control, as described in Chapter 8, designated 'neglected tropical diseases' such as yaws, dengue fever, leishmaniasis, trachoma, schistosomiasis and Chagas' disease re-emerged towards the end of the twentieth century, or were newly emergent in areas thought no longer at risk, largely due to the deterioration in economic conditions either locally or nationally.

Ecological and economic marginalization has also generated situations somewhat analogous to those experienced in the early days of European tropical medicine, bringing about new relations between humans and pathogens in circumstances of ecological stress such as those experienced in Eastern Congo and the Great Lakes region of Africa. This has led to a new research focus on emerging diseases. Because of conflict, refugee situations, global economic reversals, and the resurgence of poverty and marginalization of both urban and rural communities in areas of the global South, diseases once thought under control in specific areas of the globe are now seen as potentially major (and largely neglected) global health issues.

Exercise 11.3

Read the following excerpt on the extension of outpatient leprosy control in Bali, Indonesia, and then answer the questions that follow.

Note: DDS (diaminodiphenylsulphone or dapsone) was the front-line treatment for leprosy. Sulphetrone was a derivative, metabolized as dapsone in the body.

'Transport:
All available forms of transport are used by those attending to the patients in the clinics. The Government has provided a jeep and two motor cycles which are used to visit the more distant places in the mountains. Other workers are using authorised bicycles, a number of which are supplied by UNICEF and by The Mission to Lepers. Yet others use the buses or the local hospital jeep. Petrol and maintenance is met by Government grants with some assistance from The Mission to Lepers.

Two new areas were opened up during 1960, one of them being a small island 20 miles off the coast and reached only by outrigger canoe. This island is mountainous without any roads so visiting means a 60-mile trek, with only bare boards as a bed at night, and plain rice without meat or vegetables for meals. However in three special tours undertaken either by the doctor and the male nurse 75 new patients were found …

Propaganda and Public Opinion:
Dr Reed reports "Almost a medico-social revolution has taken place in the attitude of the community towards patients and their illness owing to the remarkable effect of DDS in preventing hideous deformities, which are surely the main cause of the worldwide fear of the illness. This means that it is now rare for a patient to be hounded out of his occupation. Even those with pre-treatment deformities have learnt to compensate for these in a remarkable way so that to all intents and purposes all our out-patients are employable, and all but a very few lazy ones do in fact perform traditional family and community duties."

In fact, recently a new problem has arisen. Attendances in a widespread area suddenly fell, the reason being that the patient had been included in the village work list for communal rice gathering. One of these villages was fanatical in its attitude to the illness only a few years ago …

WHO Survey:

During 1960 Dr Reed helped organise a WHO "Pilot Project" in return for which he was provided with free supplies of DDS and the use of a station wagon. Three erstwhile yaws campaign workers were specially trained to detect the early signs of leprosy. In the course of the year 73,000 persons were examined, amongst whom 24 new leprosy cases were found . . .

Supplies of Sulphetrone from B. W. & Co., of Ciba 1906 from Ciba, of Etisul from I.C.I. are gratefully acknowledged, as well as the support of the Head of the Bali Health Department, of UNICEF and of The Mission to Lepers.'

(Fraser, 1961, pp. 203–7)

1 What problems were faced in delivering health care in the area described?

2 What types of expatriate body collaborated in delivering health care and what did they provide?

Feedback

1 The most significant problems faced by leprosy control workers in Bali at this time were logistical, largely pertaining to the difficulty in ensuring complete coverage of the island. The excerpt describes the challenges faced in reaching the most remote areas, including mountain and offshore island zones. A considerable number of out-reach workers were mobilized, with a variety of means of transportation, all of which had to be paid for and maintained, and many of which had to be fuelled.

2 The expatriate bodies mentioned by the extract include UNICEF, the Mission for Lepers (a Christian medical charity), as well as Indonesian Government grants (by way of the Bali Health Department). You may also have noticed the presence of pharmaceutical manufacturers such as CIBA and ICI. Whether the pharmaceutical manufacturers were directly responsible for the provision of all drugs, or whether UNICEF acted as brokers and providers (as elsewhere in the world of leprosy control) is uncertain, but the role of these companies in research and development is acknowledged. From this list, we can begin to appreciate the diversity of input and forms of strategic partnership that were already beginning to evolve in the late 1950s and early 1960s.

Primary health care and the goal of 'health for all'

The Conference strongly reaffirms that health, which is a state of complete physical, mental, and social wellbeing, and not merely the absence of disease or infirmity, is a fundamental human right and that the attainment of the highest possible level of health is a most important world-wide social goal whose realization requires the action of many other social and economic sectors in addition to the health sector.

(Alma-Ata Declaration, 1978)

Many factors contributed to the vision of primary health care that emerged in post-colonial health planning of the 1950s and 1960s. The version of primary health care ratified as the Alma Ata Declaration attempted to resolve key problems in the political economy of health care in the developing world. Despite considerable optimism over the potential for high-quality health and education services in the immediate aftermath of independence, for many countries the expense involved in developing sufficient medical training capacity, and extending coverage of capital-intensive hospital medicine to whole populations, proved impossible.

Rural access, in particular, created problems to which touring clinics and mobile surgical units were wholly inadequate solutions. In the 1960s and 1970s, in countries such as Sudan, China, Tanzania and Venezuela, variations on what became known as 'barefoot doctor' schemes sought to bring basic health care and preventive medicine to the rural poor, and these schemes became the inspiration for models of primary health care increasingly investigated by public health planners in the 1970s (Hall and Taylor, 2003). Technical experts, missionary medical workers and a newly trained corps of medical auxiliaries across the developing world were also converging in their recommendations on a version of primary health provision through the 1960s, boosting calls for a new approach to public health in resource-poor areas of the globe.

At its most rigorous, this approach to primary health care sought to blend low-technology solutions to common illnesses comprising a major proportion of the global disease burden, for instance combating diarrhoea in children using oral rehydration salts, with programmes of vaccination aimed at eliminating some of the major non-vector-borne sources of debility and excess morbidity and mortality. This would be accompanied by a locally tailored and led set of public health education campaigns, together with a comprehensive network of local clinics, emphasizing prevention and affordability, while theoretically also providing access to curative medicine.

These and similar mechanisms for extending affordable and effective public health and health care worldwide were ratified in a chorus of enthusiasm at the International Meeting on Primary Health Care at Alma-Ata, USSR (now Almaty, Kazakhstan) in 1978. However, a variety of political and economic factors led to the almost immediate dilution of the aims of primary health care in its implementation. In the context of the rapid deterioration of public finances of many countries in the global South, and the lukewarm commitment of donors to locally led health planning, primary health care was only selectively applied, and mostly donor-led (Cueto, 2004). While influential, when successful, in reducing morbidity and mortality in some areas of the developing world, it remained unconcerned with addressing underlying conditions of political and economic inequality. The difficulties involved in implementing even such selective models of primary health care were magnified by growing political instability and conflict across the post-colonial global South through the 1970s and 1980s, which often had far greater impacts on health than any failures of ambition in public health planning, as we shall see in the next section.

Nutrition, agriculture, health and famine

As we have seen, prior to 1945 the LNHO and the ILO began to take an interest in the salience of nutrition as a factor in increasing morbidity in a population. This issue was treated with greater urgency by the UN FAO in the immediate post-war era, which also saw an explosion in non-governmental concern with food aid and relief. Across both sectors, organizations such as UNICEF and Oxford Famine Relief Commission (later Oxfam) broadened their remit from the relief of post-war Europe to embrace global development and technical assistance requirements. The professionalization of the development sector, and the eclipse or reorganization of many of the imperial agents of charitable welfare and health care is a notable feature of the 1950s and 1960s terrain of global health.

In a related development, scientific and governmental concern with agricultural outputs manifested itself in a raft of technical and policy interventions across industrialized and developing nations alike in the quarter century up to 1970. The Green Revolution in Asia, which involved technical inputs such as improved irrigation, increased use of artificial fertilizers to alter soil chemistry and improve output and productivity, the introduction of new pesticides, and the provision of new seed stock, increased agricultural output in India and elsewhere, and reduced the incidence of famine in much of southern Asia where it had once been seen as endemic. Yet, the reliance on intensive inputs (especially water) and on high-cost chemicals and seed (which were paid for by increasingly indebted farmers) meant that the productivity benefits were unevenly distributed. Concerns were raised about the sustainability of this agricultural revolution in the longer term.

What is undoubted is the impact of the Green Revolution on the character and incidence of famine in this period. Once seen as a feature of Indian colonial life, and largely banished by late colonial policy interventions described by Alex de Waal as an anti-famine political contract (de Waal, 1997), famine re-emerged in 1942 in wartime colonial Bengal, India, as a consequence of failures of distribution and food marketing. The subsequent reassessment of the causes of famine pioneered by Amartya Sen led to a revisiting of the causes of other colonial famines and of the underlying marketing, food storage and food distribution problems contributing to systemic (often seasonal) food shortage and nutritional crisis (Vaughan, 1987; Moore and Vaughan, 1994; Ó Gráda, 2009). Research into nutrition, and the relation between nutrition and disease-related morbidity, also led to great advances in targeting nutritional interventions and food supplementation in the years since nutrition first became a major public health and medical research concern in the 1930s.

Commentators and scholars of famine have linked the famines of the latter half of the twentieth century to failures of governance, responsible for compounding the effects of seasonal, climatic and ecological crises that would lead to manageable food shortages under normal circumstances. From the perspective of global health, the impact of famines during civil war in Nigeria in 1967–1970 and Bangladesh in 1974–1975 (compounded by the impact of a devastating cyclone in the latter case), drought-stricken Niger in 1973, and Ethiopia under military dictatorship in 1974 and 1984 was not only in its effect on population health and the burden of disease in refugee camps – but also in the extra-territorialization of famine relief, firmly establishing the principle of non-governmental outside intervention in addressing developing world health needs. The consequent emergence of a strengthened distinction between development aid and emergency relief fuelled a donor emphasis on the spectacular in health activism and planning whose ramifications are still unfolding today.

The emergency humanitarian aid sector has been transformed in the post-colonial era. One highly significant dimension of this transformation has been the role of mass communications media in portraying famine, transforming food shortage into an occasion for international political action, both governmental and non-governmental. While Live Aid in 1985 remains perhaps the quintessential expression of 'mediated famine', commentators agree that still and motion pictures of Biafran refugees during the Nigerian Civil War of 1967–1970 were central in transforming our conceptions of famine and of humanitarian aid (de Waal, 1997).

Exercise 11.4

The following passage describes the politicization of humanitarian medical aid during the Nigerian Civil War of 1967–1970. Read it carefully and then answer the questions that follow.

'Never since the days of Dr Goebbels [Minister of Propaganda in Nazi Germany, 1933–1945] has propaganda – in his sense of the word – played such a primordial role in warfare [as displayed] on both sides of the Nigeria/Biafra conflict.

To attack humanitarian agencies which have raised hundreds of millions of dollars for the relief of starving refugees on both sides of the conflict presenting neither political nor economic interest to them is both in bad taste and absurd. Because of its very absurdity, this libel is frequently left unanswered. And so it goes on recurring at regular intervals until the most likely publications and people are found believing it – or at least passing it on.

In a recent letter published by a leading Canadian newspaper, for example, it was reported that both Church and Red Cross relief to Biafra serve as a screen for collecting military intelligence. Even more incredibly, the writer continues: that in fact, Caritas admitted openly that they provide space for rebels' armaments in the relief planes.

Caritas General-Secretary Monsignor Carlo Bayer answered this old allegation some time ago. He said: "the universally recognised function of Caritas is to extend Christian charity to the world, and it would be ridiculous and false to believe that an organisation with purely humanitarian ends would lend itself to arms traffic."

All funds collected in Europe, United Kingdom, Australia and the Americas by Catholic and Protestant agencies have in fact been spent on buying and transporting food and medicines for war victims. Protestant and Catholic agencies send food and medicines to Nigeria and Biafra irrespective of the province of origin or the religious denomination of the refugees. The relief to Biafra is sent by specially chartered planes from the base of São Tomé and Portuguese West Africa. [Joint Church Aid] has no other bases for planes. Before each flight, all planes are subject to control and inspection to prove that they carry nothing but humanitarian supplies.'
Excerpt from "Joint Church Aid Press Release No. 89", in Kirk-Greene
(1971, pp. 426–7)

1 How did medical and humanitarian aid become politicized during the Nigerian Civil War?
2 What was at stake in the delivery of this aid? For the Churches? For the combatants? For the international community?

Feedback

1 As this excerpt indicates, humanitarian agencies engaged in distributing medical and food aid to refugees in wartime Nigeria sought to present their work as non-political. Yet it was clearly difficult for them to separate their work from parallel and seemingly indistinguishable flights of arms to Biafran forces. If the publications making this link between aid and arms supply explicit are described as propaganda in the 'Goebbels sense', then the Joint Church Aid communiqué has clear propagandistic aims itself. It presents the coalition as not only non-partisan but also inter-denominational, as primarily concerned with the fate of refugees rather than combatants, as purely humanitarian, and as subject to the strictest scrutiny.

2 The Churches are carving out a specific political role and moral vantage point for humanitarian intervention in crises and conflict. While the power and prestige of humanitarian discourse may well have been enhanced by pronouncements such as these, to many observers the geopolitical impact of emergency humanitarian aid, and its oft-remarked association with prolonging or entrenching conflict, together with poor accountability threaten to counteract the best intentions of emergency relief programmes. Here, the links with arms-trafficking point towards the political difficulty of assisting in a theatre of war, and is commented on worldwide.

The political economy of health and disease

War was not the only threat to the development of global health. The oil crises of 1973 and 1979, and subsequent recessions, reverberated through the economies of the world, with often damaging effects on the pursuit of the healthy life in post-colonial Africa and Asia. Levels of public finance deficits, indices of quality of life, and the capacity of many states in Latin America, Asia and Africa to sustain infrastructural commitments in education and health suffered greatly in the late 1970s. The subsequent decade saw the large-scale introduction of International Monetary Fund sponsored Structural Adjustment Programmes (SAPs) across the global South, presenting an almost uniform vista of the withering of state-run public health programming and the return of diseases of poverty and infectious diseases only recently vanquished.

Disinvestment in malaria control was to have tragic consequences in South and Southeast Asia, where the Global Eradication Campaign had seen some of its few hard won successes. Mandatory programmes of privatization in utilities, such as water, and the alienation of control over these utilities to multinational firms, were a hallmark of the neo-liberal 1980s. Previous investment in primary health care was scaled back, abandoning the recently agreed Alma-Ata ideal of community leadership in framing medical priorities, and relying on targeted and top-down interventions in child health to achieve a small measure of what had previously been lofty goals of 'health for all' (Cueto, 2004).

In the midst of this deterioration of indigenous public health planning and capacity across much of the world, came a new and frightening epidemic of initially unknown origin: HIV/AIDS. The discussion of HIV/AIDS, covered in Chapter 6, has clear resonances with earlier stigmatizing and racialized discourses on sexually transmitted diseases and their construction in relation to given populations and perceived risk groups (Iliffe, 2006). The growing perception of HIV/AIDS as an African crisis, configuring new relations between the living and the dead in Africa, and between medical research, public health and populations both ill and well, echoes and reiterates previous perceptions of African health crises that have as much to do with broader patterns of global inequality as with uncontextualized behavioural issues. Indeed, current controversies about the origin and spread of HIV/AIDS, the emergence of new infectious diseases and the rapid globalization of disease outbreaks, and the development of drug and insecticide resistance in human and vector populations share deep structural analogies with historical processes of disease discovery and control.

In light of the disastrous impact of SAPs on global health outcomes through the last two decades of the twentieth century, it remains to be seen what impact the financial crises beginning in 2006–2007 will have on global health. The food pricing crises of 2008, leading to political unrest and increased hardship from Egypt to Indonesia, may be but an initial sign of a longer crisis in food production and distribution. Infectious disease and poor nutrition continue to accompany systematic global inequalities in resource control and distribution, just as they did in the colonial era. Much of the world's population remains vulnerable to sharp reversals in quality of life, and access to food, capital and therapy in times of crisis and conflict. The problems of global public health are attributable to more than merely geographical patterns in the incidence of disease; they arise from failures in ensuring social and political stability and resilience across large areas of our world.

Exercise 11.5

The map below from www.worldmapper.org is an equal area cartogram representing the proportion of worldwide spending on public health spent in each territory (Worldmapper Map No. 213: Public Health Spending). Study the map and then answer the questions that follow.

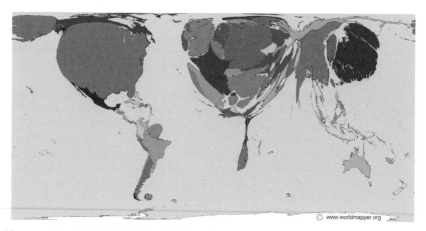

Figure 11.2 Worldmapper Map No. 213: Public Health Spending
© Copyright SASI Group (University of Sheffield) and Mark Newman (University of Michigan)

1 Can you identify your home country?
2 Is this map effective? Give a reason for your answer.
3 Why do you think there remain such stark disparities in public health spending across the globe?

Feedback

1 Some European countries with relatively small populations spend disproportionally on public health (e.g. the Netherlands, Switzerland), and other nations with larger populations have proportionally large health outlays (e.g. the USA and Japan), and thus are exceptionally prominent on this map. Ethiopia, Bangladesh and Nigeria,

among the world's most populous countries, are barely visible, while smaller low-income countries in Africa and Asia are not identifiable at all.

2 In dramatizing this disparity relative to our perception of geographical and population size, this map serves a useful purpose. Although it cannot be used to comment on the status of health funding in somewhere such as Russia (with its disproportionally large area and unevenly distributed population), its function as a gross indicator of regional disparities in spending has a strong rhetorical impact. In other words, its granularity (the level of detail it offers) is not sufficient to indicate potential resolutions to the political and economic problems of addressing health inequalities and global disparities, apart from indicating a potential direction of resource transfer.

3 In itself, the map does not suggest why such disparities exist. However, taken in the context of the historical roots of regional and global disparities in economic and political power, the emergent and recurrent historical patterns we have considered in the course of this chapter are reflected in this mapping of public health spending. The concentration of economic power in the industrial world; the instability of economic and political life in the post-colonial countries of the global South; the impact of structural adjustment and other sources of policy subservience and economic marginalization in Latin America, Africa and Asia over the past century and a half, all have a part to play in destabilizing disease ecologies, disrupting public health planning, and shifting the global burden of disease into the hands of those least well equipped to manage the toll.

Summary

In this chapter, we have explored the emergence of multiple state and non-governmental bodies, and their impact on policy and planning in global public health and disease control. We also examined how these bodies interacted, collaborated and contended in the pursuit of global health goals. We have seen how political and economic circumstances have conditioned the success and failure of health interventions, how medical research has reacted to and informed developments in public health, and how the human relation with infectious disease and food production and distribution has altered amid the conflicts and crises of the previous century. In contrast, as we will see in the next chapter, infectious disease and poor nutrition appeared to become a thing of the past in the global North, and public health began to turn to new targets.

References and further reading

Amrith SS (2006) *Decolonizing International Health: India and Southeast Asia, 1930–65*. Cambridge Imperial and Post-Colonial Studies Series. Basingstoke: Palgrave Macmillan.

Anderson W (2006) *Colonial Pathologies: American Tropical Medicine, Race and Hygiene in the Philippines*. Durham, NC: Duke University Press.

Brown TM, Cueto M and Fee E (2006) The World Health Organization and the transition from "international" to "global" public health, *American Journal of Public Health*, 96(1): 62–72.

Cueto M (2004) The origins of primary health care and selective primary health care, *American Journal of Public Health*, 94(11): 1864–74.

De Waal A (1997) *Famine Crimes: Politics and the Disaster Relief Industry in Africa*. London: African Rights & International African Institute.

Fraser ND (1961) Leprosy in Bali, Indonesia, *Leprosy Review*, 32(3), 203–7.

Hall J and Taylor R (2003) Health for all beyond 2000: The demise of the Alma-Ata Declaration and primary health care in developing countries, *The Medical Journal of Australia*, 178(1): 17–20.

Iliffe J (2006) *The African AIDS Epidemic: A History*. Oxford: James Currey.

Kirk-Greene AHM (ed) (1971) *Crisis and Conflict in Nigeria: A Documentary Sourcebook, 1966–1970: Vol. 2. July 1967–January 1970*. London: Oxford University Press.

Moore HL and Vaughan M (1994) *Cutting Down Trees: Gender, Nutrition, and Agricultural Change in the Northern Province of Zambia, 1890–1990*. Portsmouth, NH: Heinemann.

Ó Gráda C (2009) *Famine: A Short History*. Princeton, NJ: Princeton University Press.

Vaughan M (1987) *The Story of an African Famine: Gender and Famine in Twentieth-Century Malawi*. Cambridge: Cambridge University Press.

Vaughan M (1992) Syphilis in colonial east and central Africa: The social construction of an epidemic, in Ranger T and Slack P (eds) *Epidemics and Ideas: Essays on the Historical Perception of Pestilence* (pp. 269–302). Cambridge: Cambridge University Press.

White L (1990) *The Comforts of Home: Prostitution in Colonial Nairobi*. Chicago, IL: University of Chicago Press.

World Health Organization and Asiedu K (2008) The return of yaws, *Bulletin of the World Health Organization*, 86(7): 507–8.

Zahra A (1956) Yaws eradication campaign in Nsukka Division, Eastern Nigeria, *Bulletin of the World Health Organization*, 15(6): 911–35.

Public health in the twentieth century II: 1945–2000s

12

Virginia Berridge

Overview

In Europe and North America during the post Second World War years, public health developed a new focus. Before the war, it was expected that social medicine would form the basis of a more holistic medical practice. However, this did not happen. Public health after 1945 instead developed in two directions. First, these years saw the rise of *evidence-based medicine*; and second, the appearance of a new style of public health that dealt with issues of *individual behaviour and lifestyle*, rather than the broader social compass that had been envisaged in the pre-war period. New variants of public health and names for it emerged, including 'health promotion' and 'new public health'. The longstanding debate about whether public health professionals should focus on health services or on community action resurfaced. Increasingly, public health operated through networks at the international and global level rather than just nationally.

Learning objectives

After working through this chapter, you will be able to:

- describe how public health changed its definition between 1945 and the early twenty-first century
- use primary sources to identify and explain some of the issues involved in changing definitions and activities of public health
- evaluate the factors involved in the reformulation of public health nationally and internationally and assess the implications of these reconfigurations

Key terms

Evidence-based medicine A movement, in part based on the randomized controlled trial as the 'gold standard' of research methodology in health, which aimed to base medical practice and clinical decision-making on evidence of what worked or was effective. Beginning in the 1970s, it expanded rapidly in the UK, North America and Europe in the last decades of the twentieth century.

New public health A more medical version of public health that stressed a wider range of determinants of health but also saw the involvement of clinicians and medical public health personnel as important.

Risk A future harm that can be avoided or mitigated. A concept widely disseminated in Western societies after the 1960s. Its particular application within public health came through the rise of the 'risk factor' in chronic disease epidemiology. This was the likely long-term risk of taking part in a health-related activity such as smoking.

Introduction

Before and during the Second World War, it was expected that health care and medical practice would be better in the post-war era. In the event, as we saw in Chapter 9, health services were based on the treatment of sickness rather than the promotion of public health. Public health took a different route in the post-war decades, but many of the pre-war tensions and debates continued. We will now explore these through a case-study of developments in Britain.

The changing pattern of disease

As a discipline and as a practice, public health lost out in terms of status and power in the coming of the National Health Service (NHS). As we saw in Chapter 9, the new service was based not on the Medical Officer of Health and his 'empire' but rather on the voluntary hospitals and a specialist system of health care. Hopes that medical practice might take on board the ideas of social medicine disappeared. Locally, the general practitioner rather than the Medical Officer of Health became the lynch pin of health services, a further development of the territorial battles between the two specialities that had marked the inter-war years.

The nature of disease also began to change in the post-war period and this had its impact on the definition and focus of public health.

Exercise 12.1: Changing patterns of mortality, 1917–2007

Examine Figure 12.1, which shows trends in the major causes of death in England and Wales for males and females from 1917 to 2007, and then answer the questions that follow.

1 What happens to mortality rates for infectious diseases?
2 What happens to mortality rates for cancer and circulatory diseases?
3 What factors might explain the pattern you have observed in mortality trends?

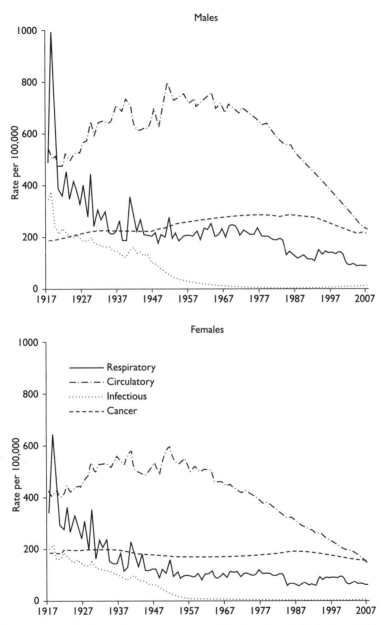

Figure 12.1 Age standardized mortality rates by cause of death and sex in England and Wales, 1917–2007

Source: Dunnell (2008, p. 17)

Feedback

1 Overall, from 1917 to 2007, mortality rates for infectious diseases for both males and females declined, with a very slight increase in deaths, particularly in males, from the late 1980s.
2 The pattern of mortality rates for cancer and circulatory diseases is a little more complicated. In males, cancer mortality increased from 1917 until the 1980s, when it began to decline. For females cancer mortality has remained broadly the same. Deaths from circulatory diseases in both males and females rose until the 1950s, after which they began to decline.
3 You probably came up with a number of reasons why deaths from infectious diseases declined. Factors include the introduction of immunization for childhood diseases such as polio, diphtheria and measles, as well as an improvement in living conditions. The slight rise in deaths from infectious diseases since the late 1980s is due to HIV/AIDS. You may have speculated that the rise in cancer mortality in males was as a result of behaviours such as smoking. The growth of deaths from circulatory diseases could also be linked to lifestyle factors. The key point to remember is that as infectious disease declined, mortality from longer-term illnesses such as cancer and heart disease assumed greater prominence.

Lifestyle public health and evidence-based medicine

This changing pattern of disease helped to underpin the new focus of social medicine that emerged in the 1950s. The focus was on chronic disease and on the role of quantitative techniques to investigate it. The technical tools used were those of chronic disease epidemiology with ideas of 'risk' and the 'risk factor'. Thus rather than direct causation or the immediate impact of germs or agents of infection, public health personnel began to concentrate on the role of long-term risk factors that might bring about ill-health over a long period of time rather than immediately. The importance of what was called 'lifestyle' – that is, of individual behaviour and habits – began to be stressed, and how these might be modified.

A second and related legacy of social medicine was what became called *evidence-based medicine*. This was part of the post-war moves to make medicine more effective (rather than reforming it wholesale) and to apply quantitative techniques to evaluate what it did.

In the sections below, we look at both of these developments.

Lifestyle public health

A key text that epitomized the change to chronic disease and epidemiology was *Uses of Epidemiology* by the social medicine pioneer and epidemiologist Jerry Morris, published in 1957. Morris had worked closely with the social scientist Richard Titmuss in the 1930s and 1940s when they published important studies of the relationship between occupation, class and health. A study by Morris and colleagues in the 1950s showed how the focus of work had changed post-war (Morris, Heady, Raffle, Roberts and Parks, 1953). They revealed that bus drivers had higher rates of heart disease than bus conductors. The explanation was to do with 'lifestyle' and in particular with exercise: the conductors spent their working day running up and down the stairs of London double-decker buses collecting fares, while the drivers were sedentary. This study was rooted in the older focus on class and occupational health, but its conclusions stressed the role of lifestyle and of exercise (Berridge, 2001).

This change in focus and approach was epitomized by the emergence of smoking as a key health issue in the 1950s and 1960s in Britain and also in the United States. The Royal College of Physicians published the report *Smoking and Health* in 1962, which was followed two years later by the US Surgeon General's report on the same subject. Tellingly, the Royal College of Physicians committee that had produced the 1962 report was originally intended to examine the role of air pollution as well as smoking and the implication of both in the rise in lung cancer. But air pollution was left out because it raised more difficult issues, both in terms of science and of policy, and possible conflicts with industry. Smoking was an individual habit that could more easily be modified, or so it was thought at that time (Berridge, 2007).

The new way of looking at public health issues also grew to encompass heart disease. In the United States, the Framingham study of heart disease was the most famous of the new style of cohort studies. The rate of cardiovascular disease (CVD) had increased by 40 per cent in the United States since 1940; new theories drew attention to the role of diet in heart disease. The Framingham study (which began in 1948 and is still ongoing) was the first to use the term 'risk factor', in 1961. Together with smoking, this study helped to change the focus of epidemiology and of public health from epidemic, infectious disease to chronic diseases.

These events also epitomized the reorientation of social medicine and led to a new emphasis on the role of psycho-social factors in health and the importance of attempts to modify behaviour through the use of the mass media.

Exercise 12.2

Read the following extract from a radio talk given by Jerry Morris in 1955, and then answer the questions that follow.

'We are dealing with a different social situation. The nineteenth century epidemics, bred in poverty and malnutrition, arose from the failures of the social system ... But coronary thrombosis ... with its origins apparently in high living standards ... seems to be arising from what we regard as successes of the social system ... It is becoming clear that in the modification of personal behaviour, of diet, smoking, physical exercise and the rest, which look like providing at any rate part of the answer, the responsibility of the individual for his own health will be far greater than formerly. It will not be possible to impose from without (as drains were built) the new norms of behaviour better serving the needs of middle and old age. They will only come about in a new kind of partnership between community and individual.'

(Morris, 1955, quoted in Berridge, 2007)

1 What issues is Morris emphasizing here as being central to public health?
2 How do these issues differ from public health in the nineteenth century?
3 What strategies does he propose for improving the health of the public in the 1950s?

Feedback

1 Morris focuses on personal behaviour and habits that require modification. These include smoking, diet and exercise and he suggests that these arise from higher living standards.

2 As you will remember from Chapters 2 and 3, public health in the nineteenth century emphasized the improvement of the physical environment through sanitary engineering and provision of drains and clean water.

3 Morris proposes individual responsibility rather than changes in the environment as the solution. But he also sees a role for the community in partnership with the individual.

Public health in a time of change: 1960s and 1970s

One way in which public health changed in the 1960s and 1970s was through increased emphasis on the role of the media and of mass media health education campaigns. The older tradition of health weeks and talks (discussed in Chapter 10) was replaced by central health education agencies. In Britain, the Health Education Council replaced the Central Council for Health Education in 1968, and was re-launched in 1973. These agencies began to use mass media campaigns drawing on psychological and behavioural understanding to reach out to populations.

The role of public health personnel at the local level became less important and in the UK in the early 1970s, the old Medical Officer of Health was abolished and reinvented as the new 'community physician' operating as a consultant within the health service. There, public health personnel were to be both advisers and managers. In practice, these roles were difficult to juggle. There were tensions between the responsibility to the community outside the hospital and accountability to the health authority. After health service reorganization in the 1980s, community medicine virtually disappeared.

At the same time, public health became allied to 'single issue' campaigns that used innovative techniques of public health advocacy. Action on Smoking and Health (ASH), established in 1971, was a good example. It used the mass media by developing 'stunts' such as buying a share in a tobacco company and then turning up to its AGM to create a stir. Such campaigning organizations did not have a mass membership but recognized that the role of publicity was crucial in a society increasingly framed round the definition of issues through the mass media. Their role was important in helping to create the conditions for cultural change round smoking and other behavioural issues.

However, these changes did not win universal approval. The historian Jane Lewis, who was also critical of the role of public health in the inter-war years (see Chapter 10), pointed to an absence of definition of what public health was really about. We will return to her criticism when we look at the issue of health inequalities later in this chapter. Others have criticized the 'lifestyle' role of public health from a variety of directions. Some have seen the emphasis on individual responsibility for health as a political ploy to divert attention from the real socio-economic causes of disease and the failures of health care systems. They condemned the 'victim blaming' and 'sick-ness as sin' arguments that were implicit in prevention. The individual responsibility argument divorced the person from the social environment (Turshen, 1989).

Criticism also came from an entirely different direction – from the 'Radical Right', which argued that government should not institute what it called the 'nanny state' where habits that should be left to individual discretion were regulated and controlled unnecessarily. Proponents of this line of argument often called attention to the fragility of the scientific arguments supporting particular preventive policies. Prevention was crucially about reducing risk to the population as a whole not, as in curative medicine, about delivering benefits to identifiable individuals.

Exercise 12.3

Read the following extracts from two writers who are critical of the new lifestyle approaches in public health, and then answer the questions that follow.

Extract 1: James Le Fanu

'... nurture, the "miasma theory" of the late twentieth century ... attributes many diseases to social factors.

The great appeal of the Social Theory is not just that it provides an explanation for disease, but also opens the way to preventing them. And prevention, as everyone knows, is better than cure. From the 1950s onwards, the example of smoking had promised an entirely different approach to the problem of illness than that offered by the therapeutic revolution. It would be quite unnecessary to have to treat, not very successfully, lung cancer if only people abstained from smoking ... it was claimed they [causes of disease] lay simply in people's lives and that most cancers, not to mention strokes and heart attacks, could be prevented by people changing their social habits in precisely the same way that lung cancer could be prevented by stopping smoking. The vision promised by the Social Theory is not just humane but also medicine on the grand scale of the great sanitary reforms of the nineteenth century when civil engineering, by providing a clean water supply, eradicated water borne infectious diseases such as cholera. Now social engineering would, by encouraging people to adopt healthy lifestyles, have an equally beneficial effect.

The rise in the scope and ambition of the Social Theory is really quite extraordinary ... But much the most striking change from the 1960s is that advice on a "sensible balanced diet" has metamorphosed into the claim that the specific diseases people die from – strokes, heart disease and cancer – are quite simply the outcome of specific foods they consume ...

Clearly something has gone wrong. The Social Theory goes well beyond the commonsensical knowledge that those who eat sensibly, exercise regularly and abjure tobacco will be fitter and healthier than those who do not and are thus more likely to avoid or survive physical illness. Rather, it extrapolates such commonsensical knowledge ad absurdam to argue that most common diseases are caused by an "unhealthy" lifestyle.'

(Le Fanu, 1999, pp. 312–14)

Extract 2: Michael Fitzpatrick

'Today health no longer means measures to develop the NHS, it means schemes to change individual lifestyles in the name of improving health – through more restrictions on smoking in public, proposals to curb sales of junk foods to children, measures to fight binge drinking and campaigns to encourage early detection of cancer

[This represents] ... the desire of a government ... to establish points of contact with an increasingly atomised and alienated electorate.'

(Fitzpatrick, 2001)

1 What does Le Fanu mean by the Social Theory?
2 What does he compare it with?
3 What is the basis of his objection to the theory?
4 Fitzpatrick's objections to recent developments in public health are on different grounds. Itemize what they are and assess how they differ from Le Fanu.

Feedback

1 For Le Fanu, the Social Theory means the post-war idea that lifestyle played an important role in the causation of chronic diseases. It is his term for the new style of public health.
2 Like Jerry Morris in Exercise 12.2, he compares it with the grand vision of nineteenth-century public health that had focused on cleansing the environment. Public health in the nineteenth century was based on water and sanitation engineering. Le Fanu argues that after 1945 public health is based on social engineering.
3 Le Fanu argues that a commonsense observation about healthy living has been developed too far, so that lifestyle has become seen as the *cause* of these chronic diseases.
4 Fitzpatrick's argument is on different grounds. He sees lifestyle public health as a distraction from the need to improve health services. He also stresses the political agenda behind mass media initiatives that give governments credibility for doing something rather than nothing. The mass media is one way of reaching out to an electorate that is detached from community roots.

Evidence-based medicine

The argument made by people like Fitzpatrick about improving health services also had resonance within social medicine. Some earlier advocates of social medicine began to look at clinical medicine and health services and how they could be made more effective. Key to this change was Archie Cochrane's book *Effectiveness and Efficiency: Random Reflections on Health Services*, first published in 1972. Cochrane had been closely involved in social medicine in the 1930s. His experiences during the Spanish Civil War, where he served as a member of a British Ambulance Unit, and later during the Second World War as Medical Officer at a number of prisoner of war camps, had a profound and lasting effect on his future practice of medicine. After the war, he joined the Medical Research Council's Pneumoconiosis Unit at Llandough Hospital, near Cardiff. Here he began a series of studies on the health of the population of Rhondda Fach – studies that pioneered the use of the randomized controlled trial (RCT). His work became part of an international movement for evidence-based medicine. This had its advocates in the United States and Canada and was also important in the study of health services in the Netherlands. The focus was on the methodology of the randomized controlled trial, which became seen as the 'gold standard' of quantitative research. It led eventually to the establishment of the Cochrane Centre and initiatives in the 1980s and 1990s in the UK such as the setting up of the NHS Research and Development initiative with an NHS Research Director. Evidence-based medicine became an international movement.

Exercise 12.4

The following extract is from Archie Cochrane's book *Effectiveness and Efficiency: Random Reflections on Health Services*, first published in 1972. Read through the extract and then answer the questions that follow.

'I once asked a worker at a crematorium, who had a curiously contented look on his face, what he found so satisfying about his work. He replied that what fascinated him was the way in which so much went in and so little came out. I thought of advising him to get a job in the NHS, it might have increased his job satisfaction, but decided against it ... This is perhaps an unfair introduction to a serious and interesting problem, the input/output problem of the NHS, but it makes the right point in one respect. There are three different types of output from the NHS, though they do, of course, overlap. There is the social output in which the most important factor is the freedom from worry about the cost of medical treatment and care. Another factor is the increased equality between social classes and between different parts of the country ... the third type of output, the "cure" or "therapeutic output" ... I suspect there is a gross discrepancy between input and output in this sphere which needs investigating, and for which the information is beginning to become available ... The basic idea, like most good things, is very simple. The RCT approaches the problem of the comparability of ... two groups ... This idea is not to worry about the characteristics of the patients, but to be sure that the division of the patients into two groups is done by some method independent of human choice ... the characteristics of the patients are randomized between the two groups, and it is possible to test the hypothesis that one treatment is better than another and express the results in the form of the probability of the differences found being due to chance or not ... There will be a marked reduction in the use of ineffective remedies and of effective remedies used inefficiently. The cost of diagnostic tests will be much reduced partly by automation and partly by concentrating on tests that lead through diagnosis to effective action.'

(Cochrane, 1972, pp. 12, 22, 84)

1 What does Cochrane see as the good aspects of health care under the NHS that do not require evaluation?
2 What aspects of medical care do need attention and how?
3 What does he see as the end result?

Feedback

1 Cochrane was an advocate of social medicine. He supports the way in which the NHS provides health care, which is free at the point of need and does not have payment connected with it. He also sees it as a form of social engineering that gives equal treatment to all. It also provides a national means of equalizing treatment between different areas of the country. This was a topic that was much discussed in the 1970s and is still discussed today in terms of the 'post code lottery' in access to

medicines. More recently, institutions such as the National Institute for Health and Clinical Excellence (NICE) have been set up to equalize such access.

2 Cochrane considers that the end products of treatment, its outcomes, are not subject to evaluation, but that they should be. He uses the language of efficiency alongside the emphasis on social justice in the other part of his text. This is more of a business model.

3 He sees the end product as a more rational form of health care with better outcomes for the patient. He also places faith in 'automation' (what we might now call computer-based applications), and in testing and screening. The rise of screening as a form of preventive activity was notable in the 1970s.

Health promotion, new public health and primary health care as national and international movements from the 1970s

Alongside lifestyle, a broader approach to health began to emerge, termed 'health promotion'. This had contextual roots in common with lifestyle public health. The historian Charles Webster and health promotion specialist Jeff French have pointed out that social medicine had been an international movement, with influence in the United States and in the post-war WHO (Webster and French, 2002). A radical critique of medicine gathered pace in the 1970s, with a number of different proponents. These ranged from Thomas McKeown, a social medicine academic, who emphasized the role of structural factors such as improved nutrition and living standards rather than high-tech medicine in securing better health (an issue we return to in the final chapter of the book); Cochrane's writings; and the writings of Ivan Illich and Thomas Szasz. The shortcomings of models of health based only on health services – in particular hospital-based services – became apparent especially in developing countries. Allied with this was a realization of the rising costs of such models of health care and the impact of the oil price rise imposed by the Organization of Petroleum Exporting Countries (OPEC) at the end of 1973, which had major consequences for Western economies. This was a period when the confident post-war consensus about health services and the health of the public began to fragment. Faith in high-tech medicine dissipated and it was no longer possible to envisage ever-expanding expenditure on health services.

For public health, we will now examine two sets of key developments: (1) primary health care and (2) health promotion/new public health.

Primary health care

Allied to health promotion but also separate from it was a new emphasis on primary health care (PHC). As we saw in Chapter 11, this had particular influence in the global South. The primary health care movement was different from health promotion because it focused on disease and to some degree on services. In the years immediately after the Declaration of Alma Ata (1978), it also became mired in debates between proponents of different approaches. A debate between universal and selective primary health care divided the field, allied to a debate about whether primary health care should be a vertical or horizontal movement. What this meant was a narrowing of focus to particular conditions or groups rather than the broader focus originally envisaged. The historian Marcos Cueto comments 'The term [selective PHC] meant a package of low-cost technical interventions to tackle the main disease problems of poor countries' (Cueto, 2004). The package became known as GOBI, comprising four main interventions: Growth monitoring, Oral re-hydration techniques, Breast feeding and Immunization. These were easy to monitor and attracted the support of UNICEF, a UN agency that stressed the need to do the best with finite resources and short-term political opportunities. This narrower focus was tied into the funding priorities of major international health donors, which (as we saw in Chapter 11) were beginning to have increasing influence in the health area. The debate had echoes of the critique of public health in the nineteenth century (explored in Chapter 3) and was also echoed in the UK at the same time in the debates round the Black Report and how to deal with health inequalities, which are discussed below. It embodied the tension between those who argued the need for an overall political response and those who saw the recourse to technical solutions as offering a more feasible way forward.

Health promotion

Health promotion, which emerged during the 1970s and 1980s, came initially with a 'Canadian European' focus (McQueen, 2008). Canada was a central initial location of health promotion with the publication of the Lalonde Report, *A New Perspective on the Health of Canadians*, in 1974. Lalonde, who was the Canadian Minister of Health, stressed a non-medical approach and the inadequacies of primary health care provision. Behaviour was important but this was behaviour at both individual and corporate levels. Particular countries also developed policy documents in the 1970s, such as Britain's *Prevention and Health: Everybody's Business* (Department of Health, 1976), which was discussed in Chapter 2. The work of WHO and its regional organizations was important in taking health promotion forward. The Pan American Health Organization (PAHO) and WHO's European regional organization (WHO-Euro) played key roles. The WHO had adopted the slogan of 'Health for All by the year 2000' in 1981. In 1984, WHO-Euro adopted thirty-eight targets to achieve that goal. The WHO regional committee had taken the stance that lifestyles needed to be understood as collective behaviours rooted in social context. This was an approach that moved beyond health care to social reform and equity.

In 1986, at a conference held in Ottawa, under the leadership of WHO and with strong support from its charismatic Director General Halfdan Mahler, the Charter for Health Promotion was adopted. The Ottawa Charter moved the focus of public health from disease prevention to 'capacity building for health'.

Exercise 12.5

Read the following extract from the Ottawa Charter, and then itemize some ways in which this vision of public health differs from those you read about in Chapters 2, 3 and 10 in particular.

'The fundamental conditions and resources for health are peace, shelter, education, food, income, a stable ecosystem, sustainable resources, social justice and equity. Improvement in health requires a secure foundation in these basic prerequisites.'

(WHO, 1986)

Feedback

There is no discussion of water or sanitation as you would expect in the nineteenth-century vision of public health, but the Charter mentions sustainable resources, which implies a brief wider than sanitation.

There is no mention of individual behaviour, but instead a much broader range of contextual issues appear. Social reform and social justice are integral to public health; issues such as peace that were not part of the discussion before are linked to health benefits.

In some countries such as the United States, health promotion remained more closely tied to health education and structurally to chronic disease prevention. But WHO-Euro and its Health Education Unit, led by the sociologist Ilona Kickbusch, developed the 'settings' approach, which focused on creating networks. The Regional Office began to work with local authorities, cities, universities, organizations, hospitals and schools. This was what Kickbusch called an 'international learning process' (Kickbusch, 2003). In 1987, the Healthy Cities project was launched explicitly to bypass national ministries and aimed at localizing health promotion, building a strong lobby at the local level (Peterson and Lupton, 1996). In Liverpool, England, a regional health promotion group developed in the Mersey Regional Health Authority and Howard Seymour was recruited as the country's first Regional Health Promotion Officer. The health promoter Jeff French remembered that these were exciting times:

'From a practitioner perspective, the 1980s and 1990s were a liberating and exiting time when the health promotion paradigm with its focus on empowerment and personal development began to challenge the dominant public health approach characterised by a patronising and patriarchal medical establishment.'
(French in Berridge, Christie and Tansey, 2006, p. 36)

'Old public health' attempted to subvert the new discipline of health promotion: first by redefining it as a subset of mainstream public health, and then by promotion of a set of activities called the 'new public health'. Some argued that the new public health was simply an attempt to regain control of the public health agenda from health promotion interests, who were far from exclusively medical. The subsequent rise of multidisciplinary public health in the UK saw the integration of health promotion practitioners within the public health profession and the change from public health as a medical only occupation (Evans and Knight, 2006).

Dilemmas for public health: Health inequalities

These battles over organizational territory also embodied dilemmas for public health. We can examine these through one example: the issue of health inequalities and the Black Report of 1980 (Department of Health and Social Security, 1980). The Black Report was commissioned by the British Labour government in the 1970s, but presented to the incoming Conservative government in 1980. Its recommendations were less acceptable to the new government and the report was published on a public holiday in a limited number of copies. The resultant media furore gained the report great publicity: there was a re-run with another report on inequalities, *The Health Divide* (Whitehead, 1987), commissioned by David Player as the head of the Health Education Council (Berridge and Blume, 2003). The received view of the rejection of the report was that its conclusions did not suit the agenda of a Conservative government. But there was also another dimension. Some of the leading researchers on the committee that drew up the report could not agree on what the focus of public health interventions should be. Their disagreements delayed the production of the report.

Exercise 12.6

Read the extract below from a witness seminar (an historical focus group, where key participants in an event are brought together to discuss past events) held in 1999 with members of the Black Committee. Then answer the questions that follow.

> 'Morris, J: ... the way the committee discussed it, it was hospital services. And there developed a major difference of opinion between Peter [the sociologist Peter Townsend] and myself on this, which you can treat at various levels ... The idea that I should in any way support a suggestion that a penny less should go to the hospital services that already were inadequately funded was quite unacceptable ... And, it isn't that ... I was unaware of the idea of community services; that was not the point. You can actually have both ...'
>
> (Morris in Berridge and Blume, 2003)

1 What dilemma is Morris articulating here?
2 Can you relate this to other issues that have emerged for public health over time?

Feedback

1 Morris is referring to disagreements over how funding and strategies to deal with inequality should be focused. One view was that expenditure on acute (hospital) services should be reduced and the expenditure on community initiatives and services should be increased. Another view was that a wide range of interrelated measures was needed – some addressed directly to the health services, others to the alleviation of poverty more generally.
2 This debate might remind you of Hamlin's criticism of public health in the nineteenth century – that it did not deal with social inequality. Or, it might remind you of the criticisms of public health in the inter-war years – that it focused on the provision of services to the exclusion of community action and the alleviation of poverty.

The revival of communicable diseases

Post-war public health was predicated on the rise of 'lifestyle' conditions and the health transition to chronic disease. The age of epidemic disease was over. But events in the 1980s undermined that certainty. After a period when chronic and degenerative diseases had dominated policy discussions, communicable diseases came back on to the political agenda. In the UK, outbreaks of salmonella food poisoning at Stanley Royd Hospital in Wakefield in 1984, and legionnaire's disease at Stafford in the following year, highlighted the shortage of specialists to deal with such outbreaks. The advent of HIV/AIDS as a potentially lethal epidemic disease began to dominate the health agenda in the mid-1980s and after. *Listeria* and bovine spongiform encephalopathy (BSE) joined the expanding list of communicable diseases. The speciality of community medicine in the UK was in no shape to deal with such threats. The Chief Medical Officer, Sir Donald Acheson, who was also heavily involved in the policy response to HIV/AIDS, chaired an enquiry into the future of the public health function, which reported in 1988 (Acheson, 1988). Public health as an occupation sought a revived role on the back of the new focus on epidemic disease. The report, however, was criticized because its primary emphasis was on the maintenance of parity with other medical specialisms.

The globalization of public health?

Towards the end of the twentieth century, health issues and the ways in which they were dealt with began to move beyond national boundaries. In part this was because diseases themselves became global phenomena. In the 1990s, outbreaks of unfamiliar diseases, such as bird flu, were affecting humans for the first time, and there were unexpected outbreaks of 'old' diseases such as plague, cholera and typhoid. HIV/AIDS became a global disease and others, such as malaria and tuberculosis, which had all but disappeared from industrialized countries, reappeared. So, people in low- and middle-income countries and those in the industrialized world were all potentially affected.

New players entered the global health arena. Policies of structural adjustment were pursued by organizations such as the World Bank and the International Monetary Fund (IMF) in the 1980s as a condition for repayment of debt and getting new loans. Services such as health and education, which had previously been provided free, now had charges attached. The World Bank's health funding eclipsed that of WHO in the 1990s. Regional interests in public health also became increasingly important. The European Union (EU) became a significant player after the 1992 Treaty of Maastricht introduced the principle of subsidiarity and led to the emergence of eight new public health programmes. The EU played an important role in developing tobacco control strategies in the 1980s and 1990s.

WHO refashioned itself to survive the growing influence of these new and powerful actors. Its essential drugs programme in the 1980s had incurred the opposition of the United States and its pharmaceutical companies. In the 1990s, WHO positioned itself as coordinator, strategic planner and leader of global health initiatives working in partnerships with new players. In part this was a response to the Children's Vaccine Initiative, seen by WHO as an attempt by UNICEF, the World Bank, the UN Development Programme and other players to gain control of vaccine development (Brown, Cueto and Fee, 2006). The appointment of Gro Harlem Bruntland as Director General in 1998 brought new impetus to the organization. A former Prime Minister of Norway, she had been chair of the UN World Commission on Environment and Development and had produced the Bruntland Report, which led to the Earth Summit of 1992. Bruntland moved to reposition WHO. She recognized the importance of economic interests in public health and brought these together in the Commission on Macroeconomics and Health. This commission was chaired by the economist Jeffrey Sachs and included the World Bank, the IMF, the World Trade Organization and UN Development Programme. Its report, issued in 2001, argued that improving health in developing countries was essential to their economic development (WHO, 2001). Although this economic approach was controversial, the membership of the Commission underlined the new role of WHO as the coordinator of global initiatives. Its membership demonstrated the importance of organizations concerned with world trade and trade agreements such as TRIPS (the Agreement on Trade-Related Aspects of Intellectual Property Rights) to global health.

Bruntland also began to organize global partnerships. From the 1990s, there was a proliferation of initiatives bringing together state, market and civil society organizations. Non-governmental organizations (NGOs), or civil society organizations, became more important in the global policy-making process, in particular after their involvement in emergency and disaster relief in the 1980s and 1990s (Berridge, Loughlin and Herring, 2009). What have been called Global Public Private Partnerships (GPPPs) have focused on specific targets. Key examples have been the Global Fund to Fight AIDS, Tuberculosis and Malaria (GFATM) and the GAVI Alliance. Global Public Private Partnerships have involved profit-making organizations directly in decision-making. Contemporary philanthropic foundations, in particular the Bill and Melinda Gates Foundation, have become major actors in the GPPPs. New targets have also been set. The UN Millennium Development Goals set eight targets to be met by 2015, including halving extreme poverty and providing universal primary education.

Public health campaigning also took on a global rather than simply a national dimension. Tobacco is one example. China opened up as an area of concern in part because of the activities of public health activists there but also because epidemiologists, such as Richard Peto, began to expand their research to use figures beyond national boundaries. New research, for example that on passive smoking, published in the early 1980s, used data from Japan. The WHO became involved through the Framework Convention on Tobacco Control (2005), which, for the first time, saw that organization develop a piece of international law rather than simply a marketing code as it had done with breast milk substitutes in the 1980s.

Summary

After 1945, public health developed a focus on lifestyle and risk, the modification of individual behaviour. In the UK, the profession moved away from its local roots into the health service and local strategies, such as health education, gave way to the use of the mass media and advertising campaigns. New variants emerged such as evidence-based medicine, primary health care, health promotion and new public health. Towards the end of the twentieth century, communicable diseases came back on to the public health agenda. Public health campaigning and action assumed a greater supranational even global dimension. In the final chapter of this book, we bring together what we have learnt to consider how and why history is used in policy and practice.

References and further reading

Acheson D (Acheson Report) (1988) *Public Health in England: The Report of the Committee of Inquiry into the Future Development of the Public Health Function.* London: HMSO.

Berridge V (2001) Jerry Morris, *International Journal of Epidemiology,* 30: 1141–5.

Berridge V (2007) *Marketing Health: Smoking and the Discourse of Public Health in Britain, 1945–2000.* Oxford: Oxford University Press.

Berridge V and Blume S (2003) *Poor Health: Social Inequality Before and After the Black Report.* London: Frank Cass.

Berridge V, Christie D and Tansey EM (2006) *Public Health in the 1980s and 90s: Decline and Rise?* London: UCL Press.

Berridge V, Loughlin K and Herring R (2009) Historical dimensions of global health governance, in Buse K, Hein W and Drager N (eds) *Making Sense of Global Health Governance: A Policy Perspective* (pp. 28–46). Basingstoke: Palgrave Macmillan.

Brown T, Cueto M and Fee E (2006) The World Health Organisation and the transition from international to global health, *American Journal of Public Health*, 96(1): 62–72.

Cochrane A (1972) *Effectiveness and Efficiency: Random Reflections on Health Services.* London: Nuffield Provincial Hospitals Trust (reprinted in 1999 by the Royal Society of Medicine).

Cueto M (2004) The origins of primary health care and selective primary health care, *American Journal of Public Health*, 94(11): 1864–74.

Department of Health (1977) *Prevention and Health: Everybody's Business.* London: HMSO.

Department of Health and Social Security (Black Report) (1980) *Inequalities in Health: Report of a Research Working Group.* London: DHSS.

Dunnell K (2008) *Ageing and Mortality in the UK: National Statistician's Annual Article on the Population.* London: Office of National Statistics.

Evans D and Knight T (2006) *There was no Plan! The Origins and Development of Multidisciplinary Public Health in the UK.* Bristol: Faculty of Health and Social Care, University of the West of England. Available from: http://hsc.uwe.ac.uk/net/research/data/sites/1/galleryimages/research/history_of_mdph_witness_seminar_report.pdf (accessed 11 March 2011).

Fitzpatrick M (2001) *The Tyranny of Health: Doctors and the Regulation of Lifestyle.* London: Routledge.

Kickbusch L (2003) The contribution of the World Health Organisation to a new public health and health promotion, *American Journal of Public Health*, 93(3): 383–8.

Lalonde M (Lalonde Report) (1974) *A New Perspective on the Health of Canadians: A Working Document.* Ottawa: Government of Canada.

Le Fanu J (1999) *The Rise and Fall of Modern Medicine.* London: Little Brown.

McQueen DV (2008) Self reflections on health promotion in the UK and the USA, *Public Health*, 122: 1035–7.

Morris J (1957) *Uses of Epidemiology.* Edinburgh: E & S Livingstone.

Morris JN, Heady JA, Raffle PAB, Roberts CG and Parks JW (1953) Coronary heart disease and the physical activity of work, *The Lancet*, 2: 1053–7, 1111–20.

Peterson A and Lupton D (1996) *The New Public Health: Health and Self in the Age of Risk.* London: Sage.

Royal College of Physicians (1962) *Smoking and Health: A Report on Smoking in Relation to Lung Cancer and Other Diseases.* London: RCP.

Turshen M (1989) *The Politics of Public Health.* London: Zed Books.

US Department of Health, Education and Welfare (1964) *Smoking and Health: Report of the Advisory Committee to the Surgeon General of the Public Health Service.* Public Health Service Publication No. 1103. Washington, DC: US Government Printing Office.

van Ginneken N, Lewin S and Berridge V (2010) The emergence of community health worker programmes in the late apartheid era in South Africa: An historical analysis, *Social Science and Medicine*, 71: 1110–18.

Webster C and French J (2002) The cycle of conflict: The history of the public health and health promotion movements, in Adams L, Amos M and Munro J (eds) *Promoting Health: Politics and Practice* (pp. 5–12). London: Sage.

Whitehead M (1987) *The Health Divide: Inequalities in Health in the 1980s.* London: Health Education Council.

World Health Organization (1986) *Ottawa Charter for Health Promotion.* WHO/HPR/HEP/95.1. Geneva: WHO.

World Health Organization (2001) *Macroeconomics and Health: Investing in Health for Economic Development.* Report of the Commission on Macroeconomics and Health. Geneva: WHO.

Using history in policy and practice 13

Virginia Berridge

Overview

In the final chapter of the book, we examine the ways in which history is used in health policy and practice. We will also explore some ways in which it can be used and pitfalls to avoid. History is all around us in the health arena, and in this chapter we identify ways in which historical material is used: the lesson of history, journalist history and history to make you think. This should help you develop your own 'uses of history' drawing on your own experiences.

Learning objectives

After working through this chapter, you will be able to:

- identify different ways of using history, and their advantages and disadvantages
- understand the potential impact of history in health
- develop an ability to apply history to relevant issues

Key term

Presentism The interpretation of historical events through the perspective only of the present.

Introduction

In the previous chapters of this book, we have introduced you to a broad overview of public health, health policy and tropical medicine in the last two centuries. History is interesting and enlightening in its own right. But it also has relevance to the study and analysis of present-day policy and practice. In this last chapter, we will introduce you to some ways in which history has been used in health and to the advantages and the disadvantage of these uses. We propose that history should be used to analyse health issues, not just to study 'great men' or to draw simplistic lessons. We would encourage you to think about how to bring history into the understanding of your own present-day interests or into your work in a health care setting.

History in health

Many people are interested in the history of health. When the *British Medical Journal* re-launched itself in 2007, it hit on the idea of looking back at the most important medical milestones since it was first published in 1840. Readers nominated these and a panel whittled them down to fifteen. Champions (only four were historians) wrote about each one and readers voted the sanitary revolution as the winner (*British Medical Journal*, 2007). In a similar way, when the London School of Hygiene and Tropical Medicine opened a large new lecture theatre in 2009, it was called the John Snow lecture theatre. This was not because John Snow had any connection with the School, which was founded after his death. The naming represented the image of John Snow as a pioneer of modern epidemiology and an inspiration to the epidemiologists in the institution. Another recent example concerns pandemic influenza- avian and swine flu, which came onto the agenda in the early twenty-first century. Memories of past epidemics were examined and in particular the 1918 flu epidemic was called upon for lessons. The Department of Health's contingency plan for pandemic flu in 2005 referred to the 1918 epidemic and also to those in 1957–1958 (Asian flu) and in 1968–1969 (Hong Kong flu) (Department of Health, 2005). So history is all around us in the health arena.

Exercise 13.1

Politicians sometimes use history to justify or explain particular policy changes. In Britain, politicians seeking to reform the National Health Service occasionally refer to Aneurin Bevan, the Labour politician who founded the service, and claim that he would have approved of the proposed policy initiative. When the British Prime Minister Tony Blair was coming to the end of his premiership, he reflected on the role of his government in the 'long run'. Here is an extract from a speech he gave about public health in 2006. Read the extract and then answer the questions that follow.

> 'We have tried to develop a concept of the State as enabling, its task to empower the individual to be able to make the choices and decisions about their life that they want ... a state that sees its role as empowering the individual, not trying to make their choices for them, can only work on the basis of a different relationship between citizen and state ...
>
> The questions thrust upon a politician of the early nineteenth century were stark and bleak. Britain was industrialising and urbanising. The population almost doubled in the fifty years from 1801. The poor crowded into the big cities, usually into desperate slums that became hothouses for the sharing of disease. In the late 1840s the cities of northern England received thousands of starving Irish, fleeing the potato famine. Suddenly, lives that had been lived in semi-isolation in rural communities came into contact with thousands of fellow-citizens. The era of public questions had begun ...
>
> Cholera was notoriously disrespectful of classes. It spread across the social scale. The epidemics of 1832 and 1848 killed 140,000 people. Cleansing action by no one individual could ever be certain to be enough. The role for government was clear. This required collective action. It meant property rights needed to be disregarded and land compulsorily purchased, both big issues for a laisser-faire time.
>
> The Victorians took up the challenge by legislation, then accompanied by the great feats of Victorian engineering ... The state gradually began to assume responsibility for problems that had once been considered individual or voluntary affairs.
>
> Yet the debates of the time show the sensitivity of government intervention. In 1854 there was a leader in the *Times* that put this point with brutal clarity: "The British nation abhors absolute power. We prefer to take our chances with cholera and the rest than be bullied into good health." ...

It was an era of great policy success … It is very different from today. Our public health problems are not, strictly speaking, public health questions at all. They are questions of individual lifestyle – obesity, smoking, alcohol abuse, diabetes, sexually transmitted disease.

These are not epidemics in the epidemiological sense … But the question still hangs in the air, carrying echoes of that *Times* leader of 1854: whose responsibility is it? The individual? The state? The company? Should it be a proper area for Government intervention at all? …

Legislation can help change a culture … But we need, at the same time, a more subtle approach. This is partly about providing good information … But in many cases government is not the organisation to persuade us to change some of our most personal behaviour.

So Government needs to work with others – with industry, with the media, with civil society to have an impact on persuading more people to make more healthy choices …'

(Blair, 2006)

1 What aspects of public health history does Blair draw attention to?
2 What is the argument he makes in relation to this history?
3 What is your assessment of this historically based argument?

Feedback

1 Blair talks about the history of public health in the nineteenth century and the great problems it faced: infectious disease; immigration and poverty; industrialization and urbanization leading to poor sanitation. He compares this period with the public health issues of 2006, which are not, in the UK, issues of epidemic disease, but rather issues related more to personal choice, such as smoking or obesity.

2 Blair's argument is that the issues of the nineteenth century were so compelling that they required government intervention. The choice for government was clear, even though some still stood out against the role of the state in regulating such matters. He then argues that the role for the state in more recent public health issues is less clear-cut, because these are matters of personal behaviour and choice rather than of urban infrastructure and regulation.

3 Historians (and you after finishing this book) might not agree with his analysis of how the state came into public health. Refresh your memory of this by looking at Chapter 2 and especially Chapter 3. In addition, Blair is concerned to make a case against such action in the early twenty-first century. He is justifying the role of his government in relation to current public health issues. So his speech must also be understood as a piece of historical evidence itself, and placed within the context of the time it was made.

The uses of history in health

If we look at how history is used, we can identify three main ways in which history has been applied to the study of health: (1) the 'lesson of history', (2) journalist history and (3) history to make you think. Below we consider examples of each of these ways in which history is used.

The 'lesson of history'

This is the use of events in the past to support a present-day stance, as we saw in Exercise 13.1. Health history is often used in this way.

Exercise 13.2

Read the two extracts below and then answer the questions that follow.

Extract 1

'If Chadwick were alive today, he would not have limited his attention exclusively to the health of the British people. Chadwick would have taken a global view which would include the appalling inequalities of health within countries in the developing world. I believe he would have been devastated to discover that the very situation which he surveyed and analysed in the UK in 1842, and for which he prescribed correctly, is now occurring to an extent one thousand times greater all over the world. What he observed in perhaps 15 hundred thousand people in the UK will soon be seen in 15 hundred million. I refer to the chaotic and apparently uncontrollable growth of cities where hundreds of millions of people congregate without the most basic amenities to support life – shelter, safe water to drink, safe air to breathe, safe food to eat, means for safe disposal of waste and a safe childhood.'

(Acheson, 1990, p. 1484)

Extract 2

'Should we seek to curb AIDS by legal sanctions through public health agencies using notification, isolation, and prosecutions? ... By the close of the nineteenth century coherent legislation – above all, the Public Health Act of 1875 and the Notifiable Diseases Act of 1889 – empowered health authorities to act decisively – for example, by compulsory admission to hospitals for specified infectious diseases. Thanks in part to these, typhoid, diphtheria, and other infectious diseases ceased to be scourges. This legislation is still on the statute book. One option clearly open to us is to add AIDS to the schedule of notifiable diseases. Should we?

Historical precedent says "no". For, unlike casually contagious diseases, sexually transmitted diseases constitute a special case in which the direct methods of the law have been tried, found wanting, and abandoned. The crucial experiment was the euphemistically named Contagious Diseases Acts passed in mid-Victorian times in hopes of preventing the British armed forces being defeated by syphilis ...'

(Porter, 1986, p. 1589)

1 What argument is Extract 1 making? The speaker is Sir Donald Acheson, then Chief Medical Officer in the UK, who was giving the Edwin Chadwick Centennial Lecture at the London School of Hygiene and Tropical Medicine in 1990.
2 What argument is Extract 2 making? You have come across Roy Porter's name before in Chapter 6 on sexual health. He was an historian. This extract is from an editorial Porter wrote in the *British Medical Journal* in 1986 at the height of fears about the spread of HIV/AIDS. It was entitled 'History says no to the policeman's response to AIDS'.

3 What do you think might be the *advantages* and *disadvantages* of using history in the ways these two writers do?

Feedback

1 Acheson is arguing that the struggles in nineteenth-century Britain by public health activists to secure clean water and sanitation in the new industrialized cities offer a 'lesson' for developing countries facing similar situations in the present.

2 Porter argues that the history of liberal and non-punitive responses to venereal diseases in the nineteenth and early twentieth centuries in England provide a model for the developments of policies for HIV/AIDS in the 1980s.

3 *Advantages* of these arguments could be that they provide a clear model for action that has already been used and found to work. Acheson argues that Chadwick's focus on sanitation and engineering was correct. Porter argues that notification would be wrong and less punitive policies, such as education, should be used. *Disadvantages* could include over-simplification – there could be more than one 'lesson' from the past. The evidence used here points to sets of conclusions but other evidence from the past could lead to different conclusions.

Some historians would argue that the past should be looked at on its own terms and lessons cannot easily be transferred to the present. Such an exercise is known as 'presentism'. This means looking at the past from the vantage point of the present. As we discussed in Chapter 1, this is not an appropriate way to use the past.

In addition, historical models derived from Western countries, or specifically from the UK, may not be universally applicable in other national contexts.

Journalist history: Assigning blame in history

History is sometimes used to settle scores or to assign praise or blame. People use history, for instance, to argue that there was 'delay' in responding to certain health crises. The history of responses to tobacco is one example of this approach; and histories of HIV/AIDS have also argued that there was a delay in the early response. We call it the 'journalist' use of history here because it is the way history is often used in the media. But it is used like this elsewhere as well.

Exercise 13.3

Some early histories of HIV/AIDS, for example *And the Band Played On* (1987), written by the journalist Randy Shilts, argued that the US response to HIV/AIDS was slower than it might have been. Shilts attributed this to the attitudes of the American public, to the media and politicians; to the medico-scientific elite, who were consumed by rivalries and not interested in a gay disease; and also to the gay community itself, who refused to face up to the evidence linking AIDS and unsafe sex. In San Francisco, the public health authorities were, Shilts argued, paralysed by gay political lobbies, some of whom were profiteering out of the bathhouses where unsafe sex was taking place.

The historian Roy Porter did not agree with this assessment and wrote a criticism of it. Read this extract from Porter's review of Shilts' book and answer the questions that follow.

'"Heroes and villains" history only gets you so far. If we're to handle the dilemmas of forging AIDS policy today, we need a much more reflective grasp of the dialectics of making decisions when so precariously poised on the rim of an unknown future … Shilts adopts a scenario which sidesteps these cardinal issues of interpretation. On the one hand, as he sees it, there is public health, and that is good; on the other, politicking with, and profiteering out of, people's lives – the ethics of bathhouse owners and blood corporations … Yet this reading is far too simple.

For one thing, Shilts typically reduces complex issues to personalities, and neglects the social and structural. By all means let's blame Reagan and media homophobia. But let us also see that the appalling slowness and ineptitude of the US response to AIDS arose out of the mixed blessings of the decentralised state and of City Hall caucus politics. Had AIDS struck middle class heterosexual whites first, it is by no means obvious that the extraordinary hodge podge of agencies would have dealt with it any better.'

(Porter, 1988, pp. 24–5)

1 What does Porter think is wrong with Shilts' 'journalist' interpretation?
2 What issues does Porter think are important in the response to HIV/AIDS in the United States?

Feedback

1 Porter argues that Shilts focuses too much on a personalized form of explanation that sees the issue only in terms of black and white or heroes and villains.
2 Porter argues for an understanding of the ways in which states respond to public health issues. This is often dependent on the structures of the state and the different professional groupings involved. He argues that a personalized interpretation obscures these structural issues, which operate whatever the group most affected might be. In the United States, he identifies the Federal nature of the state as important. This made it difficult to get a unified national response. He also draws attention to the confused proliferation of different agencies, which also affected the nature of the response and delayed action.

Journalist history as well as being personalized as in Shilts' writing, can also be 'presentist' and assume that our present-day perceptions also applied in the past. Some countries have used historical evidence as a means of feeding into current political realities in a different way. The Truth and Reconciliation Commission in South Africa (established in 1995 to deal with the abuses committed under Apartheid) is an example of this function; the evidence of people who took part in past events has been used as a way of healing differences and laying to rest the tensions of the past.

History to make you think

History can have a more challenging function, with an ability to counter current preconceptions. It can lead us to realize what our preconceptions are, and how they have come about, and perhaps also to question them. There are many examples of this in the health field, some of which we have addressed in this book. As we saw in Chapter 7, the restrictions imposed on drugs like opium and cocaine in the early twentieth century were not solely related to the harm that these drugs could cause. Berridge (1999) has shown that the dangers of the drugs themselves were a secondary consideration and that other factors, such as professional rivalries, class and race considerations, and international power politics were more important in securing restriction. Another example is offered by Worboys (1988), who has studied the rise of interest in colonial malnutrition in the inter-war years. He has shown that this was not a matter of scientific progress, the uncovering of new scientific knowledge, but rather ideas that arose out of the political realities of the day and in particular the relations between England and her colonies. The idea of malnutrition and its scientific definition established a particular way of looking at the issue. This stressed 'native ignorance' rather than structural issues.

Making you think 1: Resistance to vaccination

We could multiply such examples but now we are going to make you think about a contemporary issue: that of *resistance to vaccination*. Recently, opposition to vaccination, such as that seen in Britain towards the combined Measles, Mumps and Rubella (MMR) vaccine, has been widespread among the public. It has been condemned by many scientists and commentators, who see such opposition to vaccination as being stirred up by the media or stimulated by research that purports to show a link between autism and the vaccine. Such arguments have stressed the culpability of scientists or the ignorance of the public. If we turn to history, however, we can achieve a deeper and more nuanced understanding of these responses.

Exercise 13.4

As you will remember from Chapter 3, vaccination against diseases such as smallpox began at the end of the eighteenth century, following the work of Edward Jenner. During the nineteenth century, legislation was introduced to govern vaccination. The first laws in the UK were passed in the 1840s, but the law enacted in 1853 that made vaccination compulsory for all infants led to a fifty-year campaign against what was considered a draconian intervention. Anti-vaccination leagues operated in many parts of the country and had widespread working-class support.

Below we present two pieces of evidence from that period. Extract 1 comes from the text of a sermon and highlights some of the Christian Church's opposition to vaccination. Extract 2 is an example of British anti-vaccinationist thought in the period after 1871, when Vaccination Officers were appointed to enforce observance of the law obliging parents to have their children vaccinated.

Read the extracts and then answer the questions that follow.

Extract 1

'I would like to oblige my Churchwardens, who fear their minister's straight speaking may be injurious financially; but I must keep faith with the public ... Relative to Compulsory Vaccination, what, aforetime, was but of the nature of private practice judged to be good or bad as the case may be, now, in becoming law, established and endowed by the State, and thrust upon us suddenly, is at once taken out of the hands of the faculty, and becomes the people's own question.

Yea, the first scratch attempted on my child's arm with the point of the contaminate vaccinator's lancet shall be a declaration of war – war to the knife – before my little one shall suffer blood poisoning, and the insertion in his robust system of the vile scum of human immoralities and impurities, pus putridities, bovine virus and cattle disorders.

Vaccination, therefore, begins at the wrong end; and when it is made State quackery for tinkering the laws of nature, while yet its supporters wink, permitting men to go on breaking them, its repeal, as a State enactment, must be urgently moved for in the interests of the common good.

The institutes of the creator are profanely girded at in the vile sowing of animal corruptions in the veins o the young: and monstrous is the profanity that argues an unvaccinated little child to be a danger to the health of the community ... How can a child, fresh from its Maker, endanger the public health, or need tampering with? ...

Still, dreadful as are these "risks" of physical contamination from blood-poisoning and "ghastly" as are the results too often seen in the outward leprosy of the body, more ghastly far are the risks of spiritual contamination, and the results, not seen till later on, in the soul. For the vaccinated syphilis of one subject infused into another may not manifest itself physically, but morally ... it may fall in upon the nervous powers and moral life, and quicken and develop hereditary and compulsorily incorporated evils ...'

(Colley, 1882)

Extract 2

'But to the praise of the faculty, let it be known that they are **not united**. A very large portion abominate it ... I was also present when one public vaccinator said to another "the law is only intended to compel the poor!" ...

The TRUTH I now give, and they cannot deny it, while they dare not admit it. This then is the truth, that Vaccination neither protects from Small Pox – or mitigates its severity – but it **increases Small Pox, and exposes to death from it – and multiplies diseases of various kinds four fold** ...

Sir T Chambers said in the House of Commons 1871, that "Prussia was the best Vaccinated country in Europe, yet in Berlin three times as many died of Small Pox as in London ...

But not only does vaccination yield no protection from Small Pox – that is the positive side of the case – **the many diseases it brings with it**. Fearful, nay horrible, are its consequences, not here and there one – but by scores and hundreds. Consumption has been increased by it four fold. Also Skin diseases, and worst of all **Syphilis** ... Looking therefore at Vaccination in any light, in its failures – and the miseries and suffering it entails – the Law which enforces it **is bad and only bad** – cruel, despotic, and not one word can be said in its failure – except that it pays well: – Yes it pays twofold – **the** Doctor gets paid twice, first for **vaccinating**, and then for **treating the diseases occasioned by it** ... they know not how to cure it. Why do they not come down from their lofty seats, and like the Medical Botanist, – the Hydropath and the Homeopath find a remedy. I can speak from experience of the former system which I have the honour to practice, and have for nearly a quarter of a century, that Medical Botanists who treat naturally ... find it one of the easiest diseases to manage and cure. But to vaccinate is easier.

When the public think for themselves, instead of allowing the Doctor to think for them ... then will truth be adorned and error defeated. – But the **fear to be unfashionable**, to dare to stand to conviction because of – "What will Mrs Grundy say", FEEDS THE DESPOT, – and ENSLAVES THE PEOPLE [emphasis in the original].'

(Scott, 1870s)

1 What arguments does Extract 1 make about vaccination? On what grounds does it think vaccination is wrong?

2 What arguments does Extract 2 make?

3 How might this evidence be relevant to understanding anti-vaccine feeling today?

Feedback

1 The writer is afraid that the process of vaccination may introduce all sorts of diseases into the body of the young child. He is particularly concerned about the role of the state and of compulsory vaccination. By comparison with the attitude taken in some public health campaigns, this writer does not agree that the need to protect children is important. Rather, children are seen as born in a perfect state and vaccination may introduce serious imperfections. These imperfections can be moral as well as physical. The sermon makes it clear that the introduction of particular diseases (sexually transmitted ones like syphilis are mentioned here) may not just transmit the organism itself but also the moral characteristics that led to the acquisition of disease in the first place. Vaccination is seen as a means of transferring such characteristics and making them hereditary.

2 This writer opposes vaccination because it is inequitable and imposed upon the poor. Vaccination in fact serves to spread smallpox and the writer quotes statistics from Prussia to prove this case. This writer also believes that vaccination can spread other diseases and, as in Extract 1, syphilis is mentioned with particular fear. This source also draws attention to the division of scientific opinion about the efficacy of the process and also to the money made by members of the medical profession through it. They are paid for vaccinating and also for treating at great expense the diseases that it causes. The writer is hostile to the orthodox medical profession and practises medical botany, a working-class self-help medicine movement. He believes that working people should think for themselves and avoid enslavement by the State.

3 These arguments from the nineteenth century might help you to realize that anti-vaccination feeling is not new. Anti-vaccination movements have had a long history. Rather than condemning them out of hand, it might be a good idea to try to understand them in the context of the time they operated and also in relation to present-day concerns. In particular, there is a long history of concerns about safety; about vaccination and children's health; about the inequitable application of vaccination. Such factors could feed into contemporary understanding of opposition to vaccination.

Making you think 2: The McKeown thesis and the disputed role of public health

Sometimes, as you have seen in previous chapters, there is debate among historians and one interpretation of history will be challenged and superseded by another. Such debates can raise important contemporary issues, and we now want you to think about the evidence that has been put forward surrounding the impact of public health interventions in history.

Exercise 13.5

One particular example of this process is the historical debate about what is called the 'McKeown thesis'. Thomas McKeown, a leading social medicine academic, argued in the

1970s that the decline in mortality visible since the eighteenth century was not the result of medical therapies, and only partially attributable to public health interventions. Instead it was principally the outcome of better nutrition and higher living standards at the end of the century.

In the late 1980s, Simon Szreter, a demographic historian, challenged McKeown's view. He examined the classification of disease data in this period and argued that certain diseases actually declined earlier than the official statistics had led McKeown to believe. Such reclassification leads to the conclusion that public health interventions did play a greater role and that better nutrition alone cannot be a sufficient explanation for mortality decline.

Unfortunately, we cannot reproduce here all the detailed tables and explanations that these two authors produced. Instead, we provide some extracts from their key works that give the bare bones of their opposing arguments. Read the extracts and then answer the questions that follow.

Extract 1

'To summarize; the decline of mortality since the end of the seventeenth century was due predominantly to a reduction of deaths associated with infectious diseases. The diseases chiefly concerned were airborne infections, probably throughout the whole period, and water and food borne diseases in the eighteenth century and again from the late nineteenth. The contribution of vector borne diseases – mainly typhus – to the decline was almost restricted to the pre registration period and was relatively small. Among non-infective conditions, there was a reduction of deaths from infanticide and starvation in the eighteenth and nineteenth centuries and from a number of other causes of death during the twentieth.' (p. 72)

'In the preceding chapters I concluded that the decline of mortality from infectious diseases was not due to change in the character of the diseases, and that it owed little to reduced exposure to micro organisms before the second half of the nineteenth century or to immunization and therapy before the twentieth. The possibility which remains is that the response to infection was modified by an advance in general health brought about by improvement in nutrition.' (p. 128)

'The most acceptable explanation of the large reduction of mortality and growth of population which preceded advances in hygiene is an improvement in nutrition due to greater food supplies. The grounds for this are two-fold: a) There was undoubtedly a great increase in food production during the eighteenth and nineteenth centuries, in England and Wales enough to support a population which trebled between 1700 and 1850 without significant food imports.' (p. 154)

(McKeown, 1976)

Extract 2

'As a result of this strong nutritional thesis, combined with the impact of McKeown's devastating case against the pretensions of the "technocratic" section of the post-war medical profession, the notion seems to have spread like a contagion that all medicine, the medical profession and, in fact, organised human agency in general had remarkably little to do with the historical decline or mortality in Britain until the interwar period at the earliest. Although "municipal sanitation" and "hygiene improvements" – in other words the public health movement addressed by this article – were identified by McKeown as positive influences, their impact and effects were deemed to be very much of a secondary and merely reinforcing kind ... that part of the mortality decline supposedly attributable to increased nutrition was claimed to have occurred earliest, whereas public health measures came along relatively late in the day ... on etiologic grounds, according to the epidemiological records tracking changes in the incidence of different causes of death, sanitary measures could only have had at the maximum the potential to eliminate roughly a quarter of all deaths, whereas rising nutritional standards had probably been responsible for about twice that proportion ... However, it is shown below that neither of these arguments can be sustained on a careful re-examination of the historical evidence ...' (p. 3)

'McKeown would have us treat the airborne diseases as a single unitary group, which between them accounted for about half of the decline in mortality before 1901 and would have us believe that nutritional improvements, made possible by a rising standard of living, can alone be considered responsible for the large scale reduction of the group as a whole ... we find that the nutrition argument applies almost exclusively to only one of the several diseases within the group, respiratory TB [tuberculosis] ...' (p. 13)

'The critical factor was the apparent empirical finding that respiratory TB was already declining from the late 1830s and 1840s ... This chronological priority in TB's decline was vitally important for McKeown's interpretation. First, it effectively ruled out the possible influence of urban environmental improvements, since these cannot seriously be claimed for the 1830s and 1840s ... precise chronology, there-fore, becomes extremely important ... the evidence ... to demonstrate the early decline of TB is, in fact, far from convincing ... 1847–50 was merely a short term fluctuation and not a major turning point in the trends. So there is, in fact, no good evidence for TB's chronological priority in the mortality decline ...' (pp. 14–15)

'Improvement in respiratory TB would, then, no longer appear to have been either the chronologically prior or the quantitatively predominant feature of the nineteenth century mortality decline in England and Wales ... the foregoing would indicate a primary role for sanitary reform and public health measures, rather than rising nutritional levels or living standards ...' (pp. 16–17)

'The "invisible hand" of rising living standards, conceived as an impersonal and ultimately inevitable product of general economic growth, no longer takes the lead-ing role as historical guarantor of the nation's mortality decline. Indeed, economic growth in itself, even with rising real wages, seems just as likely to harm as to ben-efit the nation's health ... Fallible, blundering, but purposive human agency is returned to centre stage in this account of the mortality decline.' (pp. 34–5)

(Szreter, 1988)

1 What is McKeown arguing in Extract 1?
2 What is Szreter arguing in Extract 2?
3 Using the extract from Szreter's paper, can you suggest what some of the current implications of this debate might be?

Feedback

1 McKeown argues that the modern mortality decline did not result from changing dis-ease virulence or medical technologies. Reduced exposure by sanitary intervention played some part, but it was mainly due to better nutrition and rising living standards in the second half of the nineteenth century. His argument about nutrition is an argu-ment by exclusion – after excluding other factors, this was the only explanation left.

2 Szreter looks in depth at the reasons McKeown gives for coming to this conclusion and focuses on the role of respiratory tuberculosis. He disputes, through re-examination of the statistics, that TB was first to decline and that the large group of airborne diseases was not as significant as McKeown had claimed in the chronology of the decline of mortality. This meant a reinstatement of the classic hygiene diseases amenable to improvement in sanitation and a reassessment of the role of public health.

3 This controversy in history has present-day implications. As you will note from Szreter's final comments, the McKeown thesis could be used to argue that improvements in sanitation and health infrastructures are not necessary and that stimulating economic growth could be sufficient. In fact, the McKeown thesis was used in this way in the 1980s in helping to form funding strategies and government health policies in developing countries. Szreter's argument reintroduces the importance of state activity (as a major driver of environmental improvements, for instance) rather than placing stress alone on the role of the market to drive improvements in public health.

You can see from this clash of interpretation over a central public health issue, the importance that historical work can have in the policy sphere.

Exercise 13.6: Do it yourself

In this final exercise, we would like you to think of a health issue in which you have an interest and how you would go about bringing history into consideration of it. It could be, for example, the proposed closure of a local hospital, the reorganization of services in your area or the introduction of a public health intervention.

Itemize the steps you would take in designing this historical project:

1 Where would you begin your research? What kinds of sources might you collect?
2 How would you interpret these sources? What other kinds of material might you need?
3 How would you write up your findings? What would you do with them?

Feedback

1 You might begin your research by thinking about the kinds of sources you could use to find out more about the history of your chosen issue. You could collect newspaper articles, medical journals, books and other written material on the topic. You might also go to local or national archives of state bodies or voluntary organizations to examine their correspondence and internal reports on the matter. If it is a recent issue, you might identify some 'key informants' who would be willing to speak to you and conduct some oral history interviews. You would need to get their permission for using the interview transcripts afterwards.

2 You could interpret these sources by examining each one and seeing what its origin was, who wrote or published it and what its bias might be. Look back to the section about historical methods in Chapter 1 to remind yourself about how to do this. You would then be able to assess each source against your other sources to arrive at an interpretation of the issue. You would also want to explore the broader context of your topic through reading some secondary sources. For example, if you are

researching your local hospital, you would want to read about the history of hospitals in general and of the development of the health service in your country. All this can be used as background to inform your history.

3 You could write the history as an article, or a book or booklet. Depending on the purpose of your research, you might want to get this published or put it on the website of the organization you are researching. You might like to talk to local journalists about your research and get some discussion of it in the media.

Summary

So doing historical research is not just a question of 'uncovering the facts' as a kind of historical detective story, but of discovering and examining evidence and then of presenting that evidence in a coherent analytical form. History is both a body of knowledge and an area of disputed and changing interpretation. It is not simply the written record of the past, but an argument about the past, which can be relevant to the present (Berridge, 2010). We have shown in this chapter how there are many uses of history both in policy and in practice. Having completed this book, you will be better equipped to bring history into your thinking and your practice in health matters.

References and further reading

Acheson ED (1990) Edwin Chadwick and the world we live in, *The Lancet*, 336(8729): 1482–5.

Berridge V (1999) *Opium and the People: Opiate Use and Drug Control Policy in Nineteenth and Early Twentieth Century England* (expanded 2nd edn). London: Free Association Books.

Berridge V (2008) History matters? History's role in health policy making, *Medical History*, 52: 311–26 (also available at: www.historyandpolicy.org).

Berridge V (2010) Thinking in time: Does health policy need history as evidence?, *The Lancet*, 375(9717): 798–9.

Blair T (2006) Speech on healthy living, 26 July. Available at: www.number-10.gov.uk/output/page9921.asp (accessed 19 May 2008).

British Medical Journal (2007) Sanitation or sanitary revolution, *British Medical Journal*, 334(7585): 111.

Colley, Archdeacon (1882) *Vaccination: A Moral Evil; a Physical Curse; and a Psychological Wrong.* Leicester: Publisher unknown.

Department of Health (2005) *UK Health Department's Influenza Pandemic Contingency Plan.* London: Department of Health.

McKeown T (1976) *The Modern Rise of Population.* London: Edward Arnold.

Porter R (1986) History says no to the policeman's response to AIDS, *British Medical Journal*, 293(6562): 1589–90.

Porter R (1988) Epidemic of fear, *New Society*, 4 March, pp. 24–5.

Scott B (1870s) *Vaccination Weighed in the Balances of Reason, Humanity, Health, Truth and Common Sense and Found Wanting.* Liverpool: Woolard.

Shilts R (1987) *And the Band Played On: Politics, People and the AIDS Epidemic.* New York: St. Martin's Press.

Szreter S (1988) The importance of social intervention in Britain's mortality decline c. 1850–1914: A re-interpretation of the role of public health, *Social History of Medicine*, 1: 1–37.

Worboys M (1988) The discovery of colonial malnutrition between the wars, in Arnold D (ed) *Imperial Medicine and Indigenous Societies* (pp. 208–225). Manchester: Manchester University Press.

Index

Page numbers in *italics* refer to figures and tables.

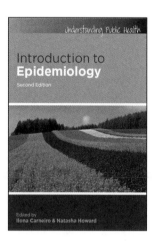

INTRODUCTION TO EPIDEMIOLOGY
Second Edition

Ilona Carneiro and Natasha Howard

9780335244614 (Paperback)
September 2011

eBook also available

This popular book introduces the principles, methods and application of epidemiology for improving health and survival. It assists readers in applying basic epidemiological methods to measure health outcomes, identifying risk factors for a negative outcome, and evaluating health interventions and health services.

The book also helps to distinguish between strong and poor epidemiological evidence; an ability that is fundamental to promoting evidence-based health care.

Key features:

- A broad range of examples and activities covering a range of contemporary health issues including obesity, mental health and cervical cancer
- New chapter on study design and data handling
- Updated and additional exercises for self-testing

www.openup.co.uk

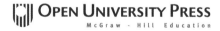

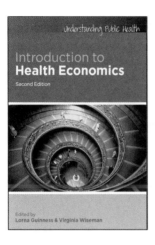

INTRODUCTION TO HEALTH ECONOMICS
Second Edition

Lorna Guinness and Virginia Wiseman

9780335243563 (Paperback)
September 2011

eBook also available

This practical text offers the ideal introduction to the economic techniques used in public health and is accessible enough for those who have no or limited knowledge of economics. Written in a user-friendly manner, the book covers key economic principles, such as supply and demand, healthcare markets, healthcare finance and economic evaluation.

Key features:

- Extensive use of global examples from low, middle and high income countries, real case studies and exercises to facilitate the understanding of economic concepts
- A greater emphasis on the practical application of economic theories and concepts to the formulation of health policy
- New chapters on macroeconomics, globalization and health and provider payments

www.openup.co.uk

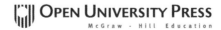 **OPEN UNIVERSITY PRESS**
McGraw - Hill Education

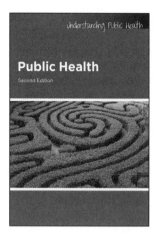

ISSUES IN PUBLIC HEALTH
Second Edition

Fiona Sim and Martin McKee

9780335244225 (Paperback)
September 2011

eBook also available

What is public health and why is it important? By looking at the foundations of public health, its historical evolution, the themes that underpin public health and the increasing importance of globalization, this book provides thorough answers to these two important questions.

Written by experts in the field, the book discusses the core issues of modern public health, such as tackling vested interests head on, empowering people so they can make healthy decisions, and recognising the political nature of the issues. The new edition has been updated to identify good modern public health practice, evolving from evidence

Key features:

- New chapters on the expanding role of public health, covering the issues of sustainability and climate change, human rights, genetics and armed conflict
- Examination of the impact of globalization on higher and lower income countries
- Expanded UK and International examples

www.openup.co.uk

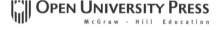
OPEN UNIVERSITY PRESS
McGraw - Hill Education